Praise for *Discover Your Optimal Health*

"Have you ever been sound asleep and someone disturbed your sleep? Chances are you weren't happy with that person. But what if your house was on fire and that person saved your life? You would be forever grateful. I was asleep about my health. Dr. A woke me up and led me to a safer, healthier lifestyle. Read *Discover Your Optimal Health*, awaken from your slumber, and create health in your life on-purpose."

Kevin W. McCarthy
Author, *The On-Purpose Person* and *The On-Purpose Business Person*

"Dr. Wayne Andersen is at the forefront of creating optimal health in the lives of so many Americans. In his new book, *Discover Your Optimal Health*, Dr. Andersen continues to demonstrate how the right tools and behaviors can help people truly transform their lives. Our team at Take Shape for Life and Medifast is proud of Dr. A's groundbreaking work."

Michael MacDonald
Chairman and Chief Executive Officer, Medifast, Inc.

"As someone who's on a mission to advance health care and implement corporate health management programs across America, I endorse Dr. A's important message. Healthy habits today are a practical solution within everyone's reach. This is a book that will change lives."

Michael Nadeau
CEO, Viverae Corporation, Author, *Working to Live*

"This book is a life changer for me. Too many years of dieting and exercising to just find myself back where I don't want to be led me to the book. The book focuses on what I have been missing all these years . . . what is going on in my head! Now I feel I have the tools to make the mindful changes to healthier life. Thank you, Dr. A."

Sue Piazza
Certified Health and Business Coach

"My decision to live a healthy lifestyle started when I was 16, and don't think for one second that it's been an easy journey. After all, I live in the same environment everyone else does. Over my nearly fifty-two years I have managed to maintain a healthy weight through exercise and calorie management, but never really felt like I was truly healthy. After reading Dr. Andersen's book I understood that there were areas I was missing, and started adding simple, healthy habits to my daily regimen. . . . I now understand what it truly means to live an optimally healthy life. If living a healthier life is what you're looking for, this book is a great place to start!"

David G. Miller
Health an ur

More praise for *Discover Your Optimal Health*

"If you think you don't need to read another book on health . . . rethink that decision! Dr. Andersen's latest book takes you right to the heart (literally) for achieving optimal health, and delivers the tools to get you there. Incredibly informative and profoundly helpful to anyone wanting to embrace a richer, fuller life."

David Singer
Creative Director, ReThink All Media

"For far too long we have been approaching health in the order of 'How, what, and then why'—if we ever get to the 'why' part of the conversation at all. Dr. A goes 'unplugged' and lays out why creating optimal health is a fundamental principle to live a full life, and then goes into the "whats" and "hows" of creating it. Dr. A skillfully, gracefully, and boldly tears down the barriers, the concepts, the fears, and creates a book that will move you, restore you, empower you, and ultimately, with the combination of education, daily activities, and choices, assist you to truly live the life you were put on the earth to experience."

Ashley Miller
Certified Health Coach

"Having failed at every diet (commercial or self-prescribed), gym membership, or at-home fitness program, I felt that I was destined to live the rest of my life as an overweight, out-of-shape man with an unhealthy prospect for the future. After reading Dr. Andersen's book, *Discover Your Optimal Health*, I realized that I finally have the power to take control of my health and live the kind of fit, fun, and fulfilling life I always imagined I would have when I was younger. Dr. Andersen doesn't preach to me, guilt me out, or tell me what I have to do. Instead, he writes as though he was talking directly to me, nonjudgmentally, as a helper, partner, and health coach, giving me the confidence to realize I am not alone in my endeavor to achieve the proper habits of health. Thank you, Dr. Andersen, for allowing me to live the healthy life I always hoped I would."

Seymour Schachter
Creative Illustrator

"Your world needs a new underlining structure of health. Dr. Andersen has simplified the process of making it possible if you are willing to work in the six inches between your ears! Dr. A asks the needed question: 'If you could choose optimal health, would you?', and then he takes you through a short and simple journey of why to create health; how to create sustainable motivation and vibrant, resilient, and brilliant life; and what will change in your life when you are all you can be. This is a must read if you want to live a long, healthy, quality life. Bravo, Dr. A!"

Kelly Rife
CHC, Triliologist

DISCOVER YOUR OPTIMAL HEALTH

discover your
OPTIMAL
HEALTH

THE GUIDE TO TAKING CONTROL
OF YOUR WEIGHT, YOUR VITALITY, YOUR LIFE

DR. WAYNE SCOTT ANDERSEN

Da Capo

LIFE
LONG

A Member of the Perseus Books Group

Designed by Jill Shaffer
Set in 11-point Minion by Eclipse Publishing Services

Cataloging-in-Publication data for this book is available from the Library of Congress.

First Da Capo Press edition 2013
ISBN: 978-0-7382-1700-0

Published by Da Capo Press
A Member of the Perseus Books Group
www.dacapopress.com

Da Capo Press books are available at special discounts for bulk purchases in the U.S. by corporations, institutions, and other organizations. For more information, please contact the Special Markets Department at the Perseus Books Group, 2300 Chestnut Street, Suite 200, Philadelphia, PA, 19103, or call (800) 810-4145, ext. 5000, or e-mail special.markets@perseusbooks.com.

10 9 8 7 6 5 4

To my girls:
Lori, Savannah, and Erica
You complete me!
Let's live a longer, healthier life together!

Contents

Foreword

Lawrence J. Cheskin, MD, FACP
Director and founder of
the Johns Hopkins Weight
Management Center

SINCE THE PUBLICATION OF DR. ANDERSEN'S groundbreaking first book, *Dr. A's Habits of Health*, there has been increased recognition of the dangers of obesity and the pressing need for effective tools and programs to assist the army of individuals suffering from its consequences.

Dr. A's Habits of Health offers concrete steps worth taking if you are one of the 35 percent of American adults who are obese today. It's a wonderful guide for those who are willing and able to make a change in their lives. However, many people are not quite ready for its message of change and thus are unable to benefit from the clear blueprint Dr. Andersen provides.

For this reason, Dr. Andersen, ever confident that there is no one who cannot make positive changes in his or her health and life, created the book you are about to read, *Discover Your Optimal Health: The Guide to Taking Control of Your Weight, Your Vitality, Your Life.* In many ways, it is the prequel to *Dr. A's Habits of Health*. Not being at the stage of actively preparing to make a major change in your life is far from unusual. There is even a theory of behavior change that identifies the different "stages of change" that most people will pass through as they move from not even recognizing that a problem exists (pre-contemplation), to contemplating changing but not having any specific plans, to actively developing a course of action (the preparation stage that readers of *Dr. A's Habits of Health* are most likely in), to enacting the planned changes (action stage), to the final and ever-so-important maintenance stage, where the chief danger is slipping back into old habits.

This new book helps you focus on the all-important mental part of making the decision to create health as an individual. It helps connect your intrinsic motivation with the tools necessary to fully integrate health into your life.

The goal is to awaken the desire and lay out the direction and choices that support health. This book can help a lot of people overcome their resistance or doubts, declare health a priority, and then do something effective to make that happen.

Since behavioral aspects (which include dietary options and choices as well as options and choices about physical activity) appear to be the number one contributor to the now global epidemic of obesity, what we eat and how we respond to our increasingly stress-filled lives and other triggers that lead to inappropriate eating are key factors that we can change as individuals.

As the founder and director of the Johns Hopkins Weight Management Center in Baltimore, a clinical and research program devoted to helping people who are obese, I've treated thousands of individuals with weight problems. In the course of my work, I've struggled to reach people who are not ready to change but really need to, either to prevent health problems before they appear or to stop the progression of already existing diseases. There are precious few tools and resources for the many people who need to change but need help beginning that process.

Dr. Andersen's book offers a simple, practical way for people to transform "I should change" to "I want to change" to "I am changing" to "I have changed," and he does so by building on small, easy steps. While this may be counter to our tendency to view change as an all-or-nothing process, change is in fact often accomplished most readily when it is gradual—a journey.

In the journey that you're about to take, making actual changes in your diet and health are some of the last steps in the process, not the first, and this is how it should be. The ultimate goal is to continue this forward movement toward optimal health for the long term, not the short. As Dr. Andersen guides you along this path toward optimal health, a process that will look different for each of us, keep in mind that the decision to take our health into our own hands is the critical first step, and perhaps the hardest. Once you make that firm decision and prepare yourself with knowledge and skills, the rest you may find surprisingly easy. Good luck on your journey to optimal health!

Introduction

Robert Fritz
International best-selling author
and leading authority on structural
dynamics and the creative process

W ITH A MULTIBILLION-DOLLAR INDUSTRY devoted to helping people lose weight, with a staggering epidemic of obesity ravaging more and more people, with a medical profession that sees the health devastation of life-threatening eating habits, with all of those forces in play combined, we should expect to see things improving. But, instead, the situation is getting worse. Therefore, we can make only one conclusion: most of the solutions offered to lose weight and create health don't work. If they did, there would be a radically different pattern.

That is the reason that this book and the work of Dr. Wayne Andersen are so vitally important. His approach does not include the usual methods that have produced a pattern of yo-yo dieting in which people first lose, but then gain back weight. Dr. A can help you take the steps you need to take, one at a time, and reach the desired state of a healthy body, mind, and life.

If you follow Dr. A's system, and if you are overweight, you will lose weight and keep it off. But Dr. A's approach is not simply about losing weight. That is only a first phase in something much more important: creating optimal health. This difference is profound, as you will see over the course of this book.

Before we dive into Dr. A's approach, let's see what has been happening in the weight-loss world.

Doctors have concluded that people are incapable of lifestyle changes. This opinion is not formed based on prejudice against people's strength of character, but based on doctors' own experiences over many years. They have beseeched patients to change their ways, and, for a time, many of them did. But over more time, these same patients drifted back to their old ways. The statistics are staggering. More than 85 percent of people who go on diets lose weight at first, but then they gain the weight back. Too often, they weigh more than they did when they began their diets. Most doctors are convinced that people do not have what it takes to change their lifestyle habits and that's that.

If you can't lose weight by changing your habits, then let's find the right drug to do the job. So the search goes on for that magic pill that lets you eat everything in sight yet look like a top model ready to strut and swagger down the latest fashion show runway. Every few years we have an announcement of the new miracle diet pill. It always sounds too good to be true. After the hype is over, the enthusiastic news reports are replaced by the latest scandal, and the buzz and excitement have lost their glitter. We find out that it was too good to be true. Add to the list compensating strategies for people's bad lifestyle habits, surgery, and exotic medical devices. All these fail to live up to the propaganda of the manufacturers' marketing departments.

Hope springs eternal, indeed, as people search for the next miracle that will allow them to eat like a horse and look like a sparrow. To the medical community, people are so weak willed and undisciplined that they need pharmaceutical or surgical help to achieve a healthy weight.

How have most doctors talked with their patients about the changes they might need? They have tried to scare them into good behavior. They have warned them about the life-threatening dangers of their eating habits. At first, this tactic seems to work. But change based on threats, fear, and visions of disaster does not last long.

This type of conflict manipulation will produce an immediate change in behavior. For the next few months, the patient will eat more sensibly, shed the pounds, watch as his or her numbers look better, and feel like a success. But, little by little, the threat that motivated the change fades away. The reason these patients changed their lifestyles was the pressure and emotional conflict they were feeling. Later, they no longer feel that pressure. With the pressure gone, the motivation to continue the new behaviors is also gone. So, they celebrate their great victory with a Big Mac, supersized fries, and a massive Coca-Cola. After a few more months, all the pounds are back. The doctor knows that the process has failed. The patient feels powerless, embarrassed, and hopeless, and also knows that he or she has failed.

Appreciate this fact: this approach could not have worked, no matter how sincere everyone was. It is nothing personal. It wasn't the doctor's bedside manner or the patient's lack of dedication. Instead, failure was built into the structure, which is unsustainable. The moment a person stops feeling adequate guilt, he or she will revert back to the original behavior. As the poet Robert Frost said, "I never tried to worry anybody into intelligence."

Dr. A understands the futility of this structure. He will describe the reality of health, which will include the good, the bad, and the ugly. But he will not use guilt or pressure you or make you feel emotional conflict to try to manipulate you to change, even for your own good. He simply wants you to understand the starting point on your journey. One of the most helpful parts of the book is when you evaluate your current health condition to see exactly where you stand right now. Like any journey, you need to know your destination and your starting point.

The other approach people have tried is willpower. At first, people commit themselves to stay the course. At first, they are successful. But, just like reacting to heightened conflict, responding to heightened willpower cannot be sustained for long. Try as people might with positive affirmations and positive thinking, the yo-yo pattern creates reversals, their willpower weakens, and they regain the weight they have lost. This is another structure that cannot work in the long term, and if you have tried this and failed, you may have taken it personally. But know it is not because you failed as a human being. You were up against an unsustainable structure that was destined to oscillate into a yo-yo pattern.

When Dr. A talks about a mind-set of health, don't think that this is yet another book on positive thinking. It is not. Instead, you will find how you can change your basic life orientation from reacting or responding to the circumstances you find yourself in to an orientation in which your strategic choices are the central organizing principle in your life. Dr. A describes this change as an integrative mind-set in which several elements come together on behalf of creating optimal health. He develops this point throughout the book. You will discover how choices, habits, patterns, and physics combine to achieve the desired outcomes you want to create. This is not a one-trick pony, but a comprehensive approach that is beautifully reflected in the phrase *integrative mind-set*.

Dr. A's approach is sustainable and can build and deepen over time. Once desired goals have been achieved, those successes become the platform for further success.

What matters is the right strategic system, because that will make all the difference between a yo-yo pattern and one that advances for the long term. Dr. A will lead you through a comprehensive, day-by-day, doable, and practical method that will enable you to accomplish your health goals and develop the critical habits of health that become your new way of life.

Dr. A understands the critical elements that will enable you to actually transform your lifestyle. These elements include science, medicine, the structural dynamics underlying human patterns of behavior, the many and complex levels of your motivational factors. He knows how to work with you effectively and as a real human being. He has had years of experience and tens of thousands of success stories from people who have adopted his approach.

Much of the information about weight loss begins to sound alike, and, frankly, much of it is alike. Dr. A's approach is not more of the same. It is powerful and original. He is one of the foremost leaders in his field and has earned that position through his unwavering dedication to helping you create the most important aspect of life you can ever have, your health. He is not concerned only with weight loss, nor is he a weight-loss guru. His concern is for creating optimal health, which often begins when a person reaches an optimal weight as one aspect of a bigger canvas. Optimal means the best possibility available. Not everyone has the same possibilities. Nonetheless, Dr. A's approach creates the best possible health condition you can accomplish for your situation. What could be better?

Dr. A is down-to-earth, yet always reaching for that which is highest in himself and his field. He is a man of integrity, yet never has that "above it all, holier than thou" style so many in his world have. He writes like he speaks, truthfully, simply, and in his own personal voice, which is fun to read and hear. He is always seeking the next frontier in health care, and he knows the profound difference between creating health on the one hand and fixing health problems on the other. In the future, the rest of the medical community will catch up with his notion that it is better to create optimal health than be forced to address disease.

This book has a wealth of information, wisdom, insights, mind-blowing charts, and truth. It is a book that you may remember years from now as the monumental first step in entirely remaking your life to be closer to what you have always wanted. You will be guided by your highest aspirations and deepest values, rather than fear, guilt, hopelessness, powerlessness, and emotional conflict.

Letter from Dr. A

> The doctor of the future will give no medicine, but will interest his patients in the care of the human frame, in diet, and in the cause and prevention of disease.[1]
>
> — **Thomas Edison, 1903**

CONGRATULATIONS ON MAKING THE DECISION to take control of the most important aspect of your life. By picking up this book, you've started on the path to optimal health, and no matter who you are or how healthy you may be, now is the time. In these pages, I'll offer a hands-on, tactical approach to incorporating healthy habits into your life. After decades in health care, I can assure you that the motivation to change starts from a fundamental understanding that any meaningful change comes from within. It can't come from outside yourself, or it just won't last.

I've spent the better part of my life in the arena of health care, the first twenty-five years in the study of sick care, reacting mostly to the expression of disease caused by people who are making potentially fatal lifestyle choices. I graduated first in my class in medical school, and after extensive postgraduate training, I helped pioneer the emerging specialty of critical care medicine. As the tenth physician to be board certified in critical care, I immersed myself in becoming as good as I could be in helping very sick people recover from potentially life-ending crises.

But in the mid-nineties, my focus began to shift toward helping people understand the importance of making health a priority. That's when I moved toward an integrative mind-set. I began to see how people's habits were literally killing them. I learned that in medicine, when you integrate all of the parts of the system, you serve the patient better. Yet that's not what traditional doctors do. Most doctors focus on one specialty and one set of symptoms and try to fix what ails you. But rather than just take care of the heart, like a cardiologist, or just the lungs, like a pulmonologist, I was one of the first physicians in the country to teach the process of taking care of the whole patient. The systems all work together, not separately. Understanding what other body parts and organs are involved in causation of a problem is key.

In 2000, I resigned as the director of critical care at a major teaching hospital, leaving behind the sick-care profession and with it, the Star Wars technology, medications, and surgeries. I have replaced them with far more powerful agents of health.

Healthy nutrition, robust activity, recuperative sleep, stress reduction, and mindfulness are now my new tools of the trade. The impact of helping a person adopt these new healthy habits is life changing. There is no comparison in terms of safety, efficacy, and cost savings.

Once people have been awakened to the possibilities and placed on the path to optimal health, the results are astonishing. Medifast™ and Take Shape For Life® are world-class organizations that have given me an amazing place where I can help others take an active role in their health and daily habits. Medifast offers healthy meal replacement products for weight loss, and Take Shape For Life, of which I am the chief architect, is a unique program that offers the opportunity to create optimal health through personalized support of a knowledgeable health coach and a complete microenvironment of health. It's been a laboratory for testing what really works. What I've learned over the years working with thousands of individuals is that nothing in my previous training in medicine comes close to the impact of my current philosophy of teaching simple, daily, healthy choices.

As a result, I now spend each new day asking how I can better help people overcome the psychological and logistical barriers to create healthy habits in their lives. Over the past eleven years, I have interviewed, supported, taught, mentored, and coached thousands of people to create health in their lives. I have written a comprehensive system of health and helped create a network of support. I am currently leading a movement to get America and the rest of the world healthy.

My first book, *Dr. A's Habits of Health*, a best-seller, has helped tens of thousands of people achieve sustainable weight loss. When used in conjunction with my second book, *Living a Longer Healthier Life*, the system's practical companion guide, I set an even loftier goal of helping people create optimal health and longevity.

I have been encouraged by the amazing stories and far-reaching success of those who have fully embraced the system. Yet, despite successes, there's still a growing epidemic of obesity and disease overwhelming the medical delivery system.

If the habits of health system is such a powerful solution, why are so many not engaging? The bottom line is that until people's desire for health is a priority and they have confidence that they will be successful by learning the habits of health, they will not put in the time necessary to make meaningful change.

The purpose of this book is to establish and solidify your desire to create health in your life and, in thirty days, to put you on the path to living a longer, healthier life. I will introduce you to the five most important things to do. In each key principle, I will be respectful of your time and your schedule. Once you have made the decision to adopt these principles, I'll help you make small healthy choices throughout your day. They may not seem to make much difference today, but you will be well on your way to implementing and living the habits of health.

The time is now.

Preface

Lori Lynn Andersen
R.N., BSN, CRNA, MSHSA

OUR NATION IS EXPERIENCING ONE OF THE worst epidemics in history. We live in an "obesegenic" society, one that is likely to predispose people to become excessively fat. We're surrounded by seductively tasty, cheap, convenient, yet highly processed food. The development of unhealthy food technology, hectic lifestyles, bad habits, stress, and sleep deprivation is leading people down a path toward disease. Current statistics show that 67 percent of Americans are overweight or obese; that number is growing rapidly. The fallout is insulin resistance and diabetes, which lead to cardiovascular disease and, ultimately, death. Dr. Andersen believes the cure for this epidemic lies in altering our daily habits, instead of implementing a quick fix. It's about intervention, not prevention.

I have coached thousands of people using Dr. Andersen's philosophy and methods over the last decade with amazing results. The simplicity yet power of putting people in charge of their health by providing a blueprint and guidance is self-evident.

This book is about sustainable health. It is the evolution of Dr. Andersen's experience, observation, and uncanny ability to help people make real change in their health. This book really awakens the dormant desire inside each and every one of us to decide to make health a priority. And then to continue on a path of discovery to become as healthy as we can become.

A recent study published in the *British Medical Journal* linked healthy lifestyle to longevity. The study examined eighteen hundred adults and their lifestyle changes. Those who moved their bodies and made healthier nutrition choices, even after the age of seventy-five, dramatically prolonged survival and enhanced life expectancy.

Are you ready to put yourself in control of your health and live a longer healthier life? Are you ready to *Discover Your Optimal Health*?

CHAPTER 1

Our Unhealthy World

> Our obesegenic world is fueled by a surplus
> of nutritionally polluted, processed food, which
> contains energy-dense yet nutritionally sparse
> ingredients. The impact is so deleterious on
> our health that without a fundamental shift in
> our thinking, we may be destined to a similar
> fate as the dinosaurs.
>
> —Dr. A, January 12, 2002

HOW HEALTHY IS YOUR LIFE?
Look around. There's a collision between how you live and the person you were created to be.

Your body was not designed to live and function in our toxic, processed world. The foods you eat and the air you breathe are unhealthy. Low-quality air warnings are issued across the nation every day. A red or yellow air alert means that you should stay inside because the quality of air can affect your respiratory system and increase your risk for asthma, inflammation, and disease. Could you have ever imagined that we would receive warnings not to go outside?

How healthy do you feel at the end of the day? No matter who you are or where you live, or even how healthy your current daily habits are, living a healthy life in an unhealthy world can be a challenge. You were born perfect, but you entered an imperfect environment. No matter how pristine the city you live in is, chemicals, radiation, and all types of toxins surround you. Most of the foods you eat and are exposed to have the ability to erode your health.

1

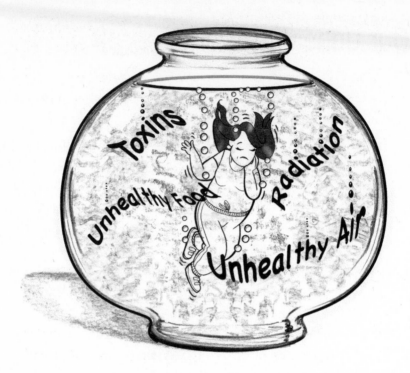

You're like a goldfish inside a fishbowl. The bowl gets dirty and a fish can live in it for a while, but eventually it will get sick from the muck, grime, and dirt in the water and die. In the goldfish bowl you live in, your body is constantly threatened with bacteria, viruses, poor air quality, and a host of agents that can harm you. This is a consequence of a technologically advanced society and the unlimited combinations of by-products of synthetic, processed foods. Combine that with the progressive decline of activity and increasing stress and isolation, and you've got a recipe for poor health.

Many experts refer to the damage caused by unhealthy fast-food choices. But the damage extends beyond fast food to even the best restaurants, which serve healthy food covered in sauces, batter, or unhealthy, fatty ingredients. They fry or sauté shrimp in butter and oil, or fill avocados with heavy mayonnaise-laden tuna fish. Even the salad options at your favorite restaurant can be deceptive: lettuce layered in fats, cheeses, and calories, topped with veggies grown in pesticides. One small salad

YOU ARE WHAT YOU EAT!

On top of all the toxins you're immersed in, you're also surrounded by seductively tasty, cheap, convenient, yet highly processed food that I like to call nutritional pollution.

Fast-food companies sell so much processed food every day because it is easy to get quickly. And it's addicting. That we live in a country where more than 40 million people are obese is no accident. In an article in the *New York Times*, writer Michael Moss described the science behind the addictive attributes of junk food.[1]

He reported that, in an effort to address the obesity issue, on April 8, 1999, the major executives of America's largest food companies gathered at a symposium to discuss solutions. In the room were companies like Nestlé, Pillsbury, Coca-Cola, and Nabisco, to name a few. On the agenda? The food scientists of these companies wanted to alert the executives to the staggering statistics of a declining nation and how the food companies contributed to it. The addictive properties of food included the salt, fat, sugar, and additives the companies added to processed goods, making them desirable and irresistible, yet so unhealthy.

The CEO of one company said that it was not their responsibility. As with cigarette industry executives, the food bosses ignored the health threat.

Unfortunately, over a decade later, the progression of obesity and poor health has advanced unabated. The fast-food industry is a danger to the next generation, as now millions of kids are diagnosed as obese, with life-threatening illnesses like diabetes at younger and younger ages.[2]

can be more than 550 calories and laced with dangerous insecticides. The eggs on the salad are likely from chickens fed growth hormones. The vegetables might look fresh, but they are probably deficient in the vital nutrients necessary for optimal health. Trace food back to the high-tech farms now prevalent worldwide and you'll find that the source of most of our food supply is less than high-quality nutritional content.

The world around you is certainly not a contributor to optimal health. It's the opposite. It's leading you down a path to disease.

THE PROBLEM IS GROWING

The United States is experiencing one of the worst epidemics in history. We live in an "obesegenic" society—a term that describes a world likely to predispose people to become excessively fat. All the pollution, chemicals, and energy-dense processed foods certainly make it difficult to thrive.

From your vantage point, making positive, daily choices might seem virtually impossible. That's why I wrote this book. As a physician, I have seen the ravages of our unhealthy world on the human body and the dramatic improvement when an individual makes health his or her priority.

I'm hoping to ignite you to make a choice. A little over a decade ago, I chose to make health a priority in my life and also in my life's work by helping others do the same. I made the choice because I'd witnessed countless patients go through unnecessary treatments. Today I'd much rather help you get healthy and thrive than wait until I need to place you on a ventilator, put lines in your heart, and prescribe multiple medications just to keep you alive.

There are many ailments, illnesses, and conditions that people simply don't have to suffer from. Those illnesses could have been prevented simply by making a small shift in their daily choices.

THE OBESITY EPIDEMIC

The largest cause of illness in America is obesity. The obesity problem is a worldwide epidemic and really should be named "globesity," because many countries are showing an increase in the number of overweight individuals. Current statistics show, however, that the United States leads the world, with over 67 percent of Americans either overweight or obese.

How do you rate? Look at the Body Mass Index table below and rate yourself.

The fallout is that over 70 million people in the United States are insulin resistant and encountering metabolic syndrome.[3]

Metabolic syndrome leads to diabetes, which leads to cardiovascular disease and, ultimately, death. Between metabolic syndrome and disease and death, doctors start patients on multiple medicines to treat their various metabolic derangements. Diabetic drugs are prescribed for the high sugar levels; blood pressure medicine, for the elevated pressure; and cholesterol-lowering drugs, for high cholesterol. Eventually, the drugs

Body Mass Index Table

Height (Inches) / BMI	Normal						Overweight					Obese										Extreme Obesity														
BMI	19	20	21	22	23	24	25	26	27	28	29	30	31	32	33	34	35	36	37	38	39	40	41	42	43	44	45	46	47	48	49	50	51	52	53	54
58	91	96	100	105	110	115	119	124	129	134	138	143	148	153	158	162	167	172	177	181	186	191	196	201	205	210	215	220	224	229	234	239	244	248	253	258
59	94	99	104	109	114	119	124	128	133	138	143	148	153	158	163	168	173	178	183	188	193	198	203	208	212	217	222	227	232	237	242	247	252	257	262	267
60	97	102	107	112	118	123	128	133	138	143	148	153	158	163	168	174	179	184	189	194	199	204	209	215	220	225	230	235	240	245	250	255	261	266	271	276
61	100	106	111	116	122	127	132	137	143	148	153	158	164	169	174	180	185	190	195	201	206	211	217	222	227	232	238	243	248	254	259	264	269	275	280	285
62	104	109	115	120	126	131	136	142	147	153	158	164	169	175	180	186	191	196	202	207	213	218	224	229	235	240	246	251	256	262	267	273	278	284	289	295
63	107	113	118	124	130	135	141	146	152	158	163	169	175	180	186	191	197	203	208	214	220	225	231	237	242	248	254	259	265	270	278	282	287	293	299	304
64	110	116	122	128	134	140	145	151	157	163	169	174	180	186	192	197	204	209	215	221	227	232	238	244	250	256	262	267	273	279	285	291	296	302	308	314
65	114	120	126	132	138	144	150	156	162	168	174	180	186	192	198	204	210	216	222	228	234	240	246	252	258	264	270	276	282	288	294	300	306	312	318	324
66	118	124	130	136	142	148	155	161	167	173	179	186	192	198	204	210	216	223	229	235	241	247	253	260	266	272	278	284	291	297	303	309	315	322	328	334
67	121	127	134	140	146	153	159	166	172	178	185	191	198	204	211	217	223	230	236	242	249	255	261	268	274	280	287	293	299	306	312	319	325	331	338	344
68	125	131	138	144	151	158	164	171	177	184	190	197	203	210	216	223	230	236	243	249	256	262	269	276	282	289	295	302	308	315	322	328	335	341	348	354
69	128	135	142	149	155	162	169	176	182	189	196	203	209	216	223	230	236	243	250	257	263	270	277	284	291	297	304	311	318	324	331	338	345	351	358	365
70	132	139	146	153	160	167	174	181	188	195	202	209	216	222	229	236	243	250	257	264	271	278	285	292	299	306	313	320	327	334	341	348	355	362	369	376
71	136	143	150	157	165	172	179	186	193	200	208	215	222	229	236	243	250	257	265	272	279	286	293	301	308	315	322	329	338	343	351	358	365	372	379	386
72	140	147	154	162	169	177	184	191	199	206	213	221	228	235	242	250	258	265	272	279	287	294	302	309	316	324	331	338	346	353	361	368	375	383	390	397
73	144	151	159	166	174	182	189	197	204	212	219	227	235	242	250	257	265	272	280	288	295	302	310	318	325	333	340	348	355	363	371	378	386	393	401	408
74	148	155	163	171	179	186	194	202	210	218	225	233	241	249	256	264	272	280	287	295	303	311	319	326	334	342	350	358	365	373	381	389	396	404	412	420
75	152	160	168	176	184	192	200	208	216	224	232	240	248	256	264	272	279	287	295	303	311	319	327	335	343	351	359	367	375	383	391	399	407	415	423	431
76	156	164	172	180	189	197	205	213	221	230	238	246	254	263	271	279	287	295	304	312	320	328	336	344	353	361	369	377	385	394	402	410	418	426	435	443

Source: Adapted from Clinical Guidelines on the Identification, Evaluation, and Treatment of Overweight and Obesity in Adults: The Evidence Report.

METABOLIC SYNDROME

is present if you have three or more of the following signs:

- Blood pressure equal to or higher than 130/85 mmHg
- Fasting blood sugar (glucose) equal to or higher than 100 mg/dL

Large waist circumference (length around the waist):
- Men - 40 inches or more
- Women - 35 inches or more

Low HDL cholesterol:
- Men - under 40 mg/dL
- Women - under 50 mg/dL

Triglycerides equal to or higher than 150 mg/dL

are not enough. Diminished lifestyles and poorer health follow, leading to gangrenous limbs and deteriorating eyesight, and medical intervention is reduced to palliative surgeries. This scenario of progressive decline is totally preventable, simply by changing our focus from reacting to and treating symptoms to eliminating disease.

HOW OBESITY AFFECTS DISEASE AND DECLINE

The excess weight around your middle is made up of millions of individual fat cells that look like overstuffed lasagna under an electron microscope. When these fat cells become engorged, they increase the release of substances that travel to different organs and negatively affect their function. As a result, your blood sugar, cholesterol, and blood pressure go up. Our sick-care system, once aware of your unhealthy lab result, stands ready to target those symptoms with specialists, diagnoses, and drugs.

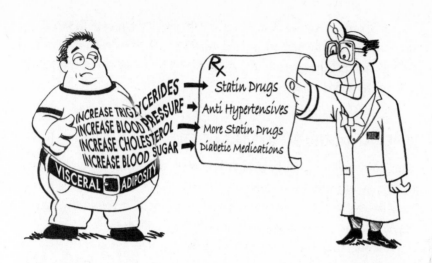

But sick care isn't the solution.

Yes, we have to be ready to treat sickness. But a better, safer, more effective, and dramatically cheaper way is to simply empty those engorged fat cells. Once you can do that, you're on the path to a healthier life.

During our lifespan, we can continue to improve our technologically advancing civilization to ensure the safety and health of the environment and food. Yet, this improvement is going to take time and a concerted effort of societal forces, which are slow to adapt. Meanwhile, I have a plan to keep you and those you care for protected.

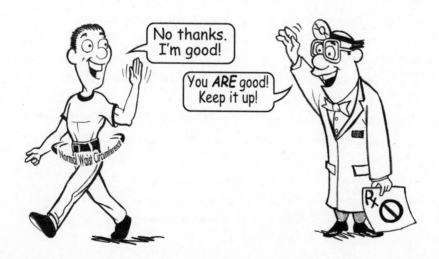

We cannot totally change the water in our fishbowl. It's too late for that. But we can do something to protect and arm us with a formidable defense against the surrounding world. The best way to accomplish this is to become optimally healthy.

THE AMAZING HUMAN BODY

Your body has amazing qualities to protect you against the erosive forces that make life and health intrinsically unstable. One example is the way your body protects you from cancer every day. Did you know that as a result of those erosive forces, precancerous cells are already inside us? If left alone, they could potentially become cancerous and threaten our lives. This is why it's so critical to be healthy to fight the things you're bombarded with daily—radiation, toxins, chemicals, and unhealthy food. Let's face it. Our fishbowl water is of poor quality. An optimally healthy body has an incredibly advanced process called apoptosis by which your body searches out the potentially harmful cells and destroys them before they can cause cancer.

This is one example of the thousands of ways an optimally healthy body guards us in our daily lives. Think of discovering and creating optimal health as a means of surrounding yourself in a protective layer. As you develop the full spectrum of healthy habits, you make this armor stronger and more impenetrable to your hostile surroundings.

In addition, when you develop healthy habits, you are actually equipping your body to fight disease. Once a disease has entered the body, *all* the healthy parts, not just one part, must fight it. A disease might mean their common death. Nature knows this and attacks the disease with whatever help it can muster. We know deep inside how important it is to be healthy, and we ignore that reality. After years of treating patients, I've been able to see why so many fail. It's a lack of desire to change, for many reasons.

You may not think good health is a priority; you may have good health insurance. Or the task seems so monumental that you do not even want to think about it, or your past results have been so dismal that you have put the notion aside.

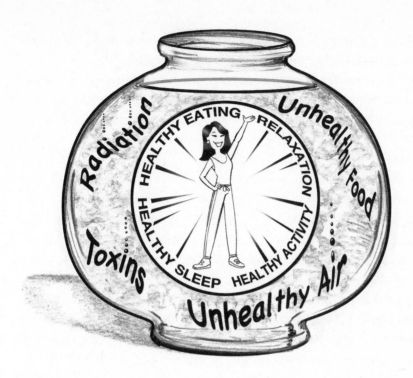

In this book, I want to awaken and bring your desire for health to the forefront. Your health should be your number-one focus. If you have a strong resolve to get healthy and you understand how important it is, I can help you. For the past decade, my mission has been to help people break down logistical and psychological barriers that prevent them from optimal health. As the cofounder of Take Shape For Life, I have built a large community of like-minded people who have made their health a priority. I've worked with thousands of individuals and families to help them achieve their goals for optimal health. I want to do that right here, right now, with you.

You probably know someone who suffers from arthritis, loss of movement, back or neck pain, or prescription drug addiction. Or you may know someone with diabetes, heart disease, mental decline, or an inability to walk, much less jog or run. How many people in their fifties or sixties do you know who do actually walk, jog, or run each day? The body was designed for such movement, but not if we don't take care of it. By the time most people hit their forties, they stop moving and exercising altogether. But that's not going to be you.

Most people believe that just because they're not sick, they're healthy. Our current health-care system is designed so that you are well until you feel bad. Then you go to the doctor to be diagnosed and you end up in a system with codes that label you. Once you've been nicely categorized, the proper magic bullet can provide temporary bandages. That's what we call health care, but does it seem healthy to you? It's really sick care.

One example is diabetes, which is labeled a chronic disease. This suggests that it can't be reversed. Nothing could be further from the truth. Those with Type II diabetes can arrest its progression and even remove all its physiologic traces. Reversing and eliminating disease is what we should focus on.

The medical system is a disease-based business system because it makes money if you're sick. The only thing less profitable than helping you get healthy is sudden death. The existing health-care system is reactionary. Instead of asking why people are sick, the system focuses on what is wrong with people and attempts to cure it. The system has created an industry, called "sick care," which is a result of early success with antibiotics and their miraculous ability to wipe out infection. Unfortunately, antibiotics don't work for lifestyle disease, which is the current battle.

The medical insurance industry is also in a crisis in the United States. For example, insurance carriers will pay for your nutritional counseling if you have diabetes. However, they often won't pay for any type of prevention or prediabetes counseling because you haven't yet been labeled. This policy doesn't make any sense. Early intervention could help prevent the problem.

By now, I hope you'll agree that if you want the best for yourself, you need to take charge of your health. If you don't focus on it, your body could be a ticking time bomb.

WHAT IS OPTIMAL HEALTH?

The optimal health I propose for your life is an integrative approach that begins with developing (and maintaining) healthy habits each day. It makes health the centerpiece of your life instead something you do when you discover you have an illness or imbalance.

A little attention and discipline now can keep you from later being an unhealthy person who goes to the doctor three days a week. No matter what your current health status, you can be as healthy as possible. The habits you develop can make the difference between surviving and thriving, and often between life and death. I'm not talking about radical one-off events, like running a marathon or destressing your mind by getting a massage or going to the gym occasionally. I'm talking about the small, daily choices that develop into habits. Daily choices. Daily habits. That become you.

The time is now. The good news is that even though we live in an unhealthy world with bad choices, we can start developing habits today that will help reverse their effects on your body. I'm here to be your personal coach and guide you through the process. I use the process every day myself, and my entire family uses it. Adding just one healthy habit can change your life forever and solidify a path to longevity. When you can integrate all the habits into your life, the results are astonishing.

One example is to add daily physical activity to your life. Exercise can increase your lifespan *and* improve your mental acuity. Physical activity has mental health benefits. It reduces stress, releases endorphins, and increases blood flow in the brain. The American Academy of Neurology announced in October 2012 that physical activity is even more important than mental activity for the brain, even more so than brain-teasers, socialization, or crossword puzzles, in terms of cognitive function. This groundbreaking information was based on research with 638 elderly people in Scotland, who participated in a brain MRI study. "People in their seventies who participated in more physical exercise, including walking several times a week, had less brain shrinkage and other signs of aging in the brain than those who were less physically active," said study author Alan J. Gow, PhD, of the University of Edinburgh, Scotland.[4]

• • •

This book will help you sort through your life choices to make sure they're positioning you for success. It will help you identify areas of weakness in your life that sabotage you from making real, lasting progress toward your health and longevity. I plan to give you the knowledge and tools to help you maintain and reach optimal health. I'm going to coach you through this process, and at the end, you'll be equipped to live your best life. The following testimony is from a woman who experienced a major transformation. Her story is an example of the potential of this journey:

What a health journey it has been! In June of 2003, symptoms of low thyroid and inflammatory disease ruled my life. I was only 43, but felt like I was 63. I was overweight, eating and sleeping poorly, under a lot of stress, and not able to exercise, due to fatigue and joint pain. I had lost my confidence and many relationships,

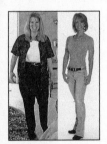

as I found myself wanting to hide from everyone. That all changed when I heard Dr. A talk about how I could create optimal health, even though I had failed many times before. It was the hope I had been looking for, so I decided to follow his recommended lifestyle approach. Not only did I reach a healthy weight in three months, I am continually incorporating all the strategies from *Dr A's Habits of Health*. I am now living the "Ultra Health Phase" of his book! My inflammatory disease resolved, because of my dramatic lifestyle changes, and I have continued to get healthier and more fit every year. I am blessed with many wonderful relationships and adventures, and my husband and I are living beyond our wildest dreams! Thank you Dr. A, for helping me discover MY optimal health!

– Lisa Castro

Stories like that help ignite me to continue talking about healthy habits, in contrast to what most of the medical community is promoting. A longer, more vital life is possible.

Are you ready? This journey may involve changing your pre-conceived beliefs. It might mean letting go of some old ways of doing things. You don't get rid of bad habits; you replace them with good ones. Then, after a while, the old bad habits lose their significance and power over you.

CHAPTER 2

Are You Healthy?

> The greatest wealth is health.
>
> —Virgil

I F I ASKED YOU TO LIST AND PRIORITIZE THE most important things in your life, chances are that your health and the health of your loved ones would be at the very top. If you had to choose between a bigger bank account and another decade of health for your children, spouse, or yourself, you'd choose health. Your health is one of your most important assets. It determines how active you are and to some extent how influential and engaged you can be in the lives of others.

Throughout this book, I'm going to encourage you to make your health a priority. The first step on the journey is to understand your current status. In this chapter, I am going to establish a new way for you to look at your health. My goal is to empower you with understanding so you can make the best decisions for yourself.

I am putting you in charge of your health, creating clear separation of my role from the traditional, authoritative doctor. Your health professional is well trained and a valuable part of your disease management. The doctor has great knowledge and good intentions. The patient sits on a cold metal stool and listens to the lecture. The doctor has important advice, but it's probably not particularly helpful in managing your weight and health. That's up to you.

Are you building or eroding your health? Maybe you think that if you go to your doctor, he or she can keep you healthy. Perhaps you have a hard time even visualizing what I mean when I say optimal health; you are just trying to survive your busy schedule.

So let's start with a blank piece of paper and find out your location on the health continuum. Then we will explore what you can do to live a long, healthier life. Agreed?

In my first book, *Dr. A's Habits of Health*, I outlined the typical health path of most humans, which is a steady trajectory from optimal health at birth, to an unhealthy state of non-sickness by age fifty, to a declining state of sickness and disease. Unfortunately, this isn't the path to optimal health, and, tragically, 90 percent of people fall into the non-sick category with their unhealthy choices heading them toward disease. That means that most of us are simply surviving, instead of thriving and creating daily habits that lead to a vibrant, active life well into later years.

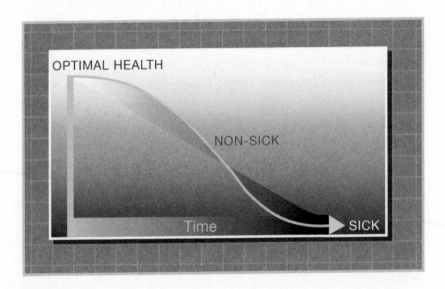

YOUR HEALTH CONTINUUM QUIZ

The ten questions on the following page will give you an idea how healthy or sick you are and your current position on the graph. When answering these questions, think about the average of your past thirty days.

Add up your score, and look at the assessment below to see your current position on the continuum.

Your Current Health Continuum Position

OPTIMAL HEALTH < 5 — CONGRATULATIONS!

At this point, you have adapted to living in the fishbowl and are currently in great health. This could be because you are young, have great genes, and are making great daily choices. You can stay that way. There is always more you can do to maintain and improve your health and the best time to do it is when you are still healthy.

NON-SICK 5–20

If your score is in this range, your body is starting to show symptoms of moving toward disease. As I mentioned, almost 90 percent of the population falls into this non-sick category and your health is starting to be affected negatively from living in the fishbowl even if outwardly you appear OK.

If, in addition, your genetics are not the best (your parents or grand-parents died early or had serious disease), it is important to recognize that your current behavior and choices are withdrawing vitality from your health account.

The good news is that this book is going to help you lower that score by developing your mind-set to move your choices toward optimal health, which will improve your current health. This is especially important in helping offset your risk of developing disease if you have been dealt a bad hand by your genes.

SICK >20

If your score is in this range, your body is in a disease state. Over-the-counter medications or pharmaceuticals can mask your body's symptoms,

YOUR HEALTH CONTINUUM QUIZ

The following 10 questions will give you an idea of where you are currently. When answering these questions, think about the average of the last 30 days of your life:

1. How would you rate your overall feeling?	Excellent	Fair	Poor
Your energy level	0	3 EL	5
Your sleep	0	3 L	5 E
Your mood	0 L	3 E	5

2. How would you describe your breathing?	Never	Sometimes	Always
Shallow breathing	0 E	2 L	3
Short of breath during activity	0	2 LE	3
Short of breath at rest	0 EL	3	5
Chronic cough	0 EL	2	5

3. What is your stress level?	Low	Medium	High
At job	0 E	3 L	5
At home	0 L	3 E	5
Anxiety level	0 E	3 L	5

4. Do you have pain?	Never	Sometimes	Always
Joints	0	2 LE	5
Back	0 LE	2	5
Headaches	0	2 LE	5

5. Do you use?	Never	Sometimes	Always
Non-prescription medication	0	2 LE	3
Prescription medications	0 LE	2	3
Tobacco	0 LE	5	8
Alcohol	0 LE	2	5

6. What is your current?				
Weight	0 Thin (Healthy)	1 normal	3 overweight	5 obese
Waist	0 Thin (Healthy)	1 normal	3 paunch	5 protuberant

7. How is your?			
Skin	0 Warm & soft	2 Dry & scaly	5 Swollen or growths
Hair	0 Thick & shiny	2 Thin & dull	5 Loss around ankles
Nails	0 Strong	2 Ridges	5 Discolored or yellow
Your digestion	0 Normal	3 Heartburn	5 Reflux

8. Do you get colds and flu?	0 Almost never	3 Sometimes	5 Often

9. Do you go to a doctor and are you up to date on wellness checkups?	0 Often	1 Sometimes	5 Almost never

10. Do you have a serious disease?	Add 20 points per disease

but can't change the fact that you are very unhealthy. Although you probably think you are destined to continue in your disease state, your decision to take control can dramatically alter your disease progression, if it is related to an unhealthy lifestyle. Cardiovascular disease, diabetes (Type II), arthritis, and a whole host of other diseases are heavily influenced by your lifestyle choices.

Even with disease, you can heavily influence the state of your health and length of life. By changing your daily choices, you can often make some dramatic changes once your body has a chance to recover.

• • •

The first part of getting healthy is finding out where you are on the continuum, which you've just done. Now you know where you are so you can get where you want to go. If you value living a longer, healthier life and want to choose optimal health as a priority, I can help. In chapter 3, I address how the medical community and the pharmaceutical companies are responding to your current health. But, first, it's important to address how *you* are managing your current health state. Your daily choices are more important in determining your health than anything the medical world can do for you.

YOUR HABITS OF HEALTH QUIZ

The next quiz evaluates your current health status to see where your current daily choices are taking you. Answer these ten questions, describing as accurately as possible your behavior or status in the past thirty days.

Your Habits of Health Score

OPTIMAL >50

You are making mostly great decisions supporting your health; by continuing to add more habits of health, you will further enhance your health.

YOUR HABITS OF HEALTH QUIZ

1. Do you need to lose weight?	No 5	Yes 0	> 30 Pounds -5
2. Do you smoke?	Never 5	Yes -10	Quit > 2 years -5
3. Do you eat breakfast?	Everyday 5	Most Days 3	Occasionally -1
4. Do you eat healthy?			
Red meat:	Never 3	Occasionally 0	Daily -3
Eat vegetables daily:	> 3 portions 5	1-3 portions 3	< 1 portion -2
Do you eat sugar and white starches?	Never 5	Occasionally 1	Daily -3
5. How many hours a day do you sit?	< One 5	One to five 0	0 > five -5
6. Do you walk?	30 min/day 10	Sometimes 3	Never -3
7. On your weekend how active are you?	Play sports 10	Walk dog or bike ride 5	Sit on the sofa & watch TV -3
8. Do you enjoy your job?	Very much 10	OK 0	I hate it -10
9. I enjoy time with friends or pets:	Everyday 10	Sometimes 3	Never -5
10. When I wake up from sleep I am:	Very rested 10	Feeling OK 0	Exhausted -10

HEALTHY 35–50

Most of your choices are healthy, but you are offsetting some of their beneficial effects by making some unhealthy choices.

UNHEALTHY < 35

You are either already sick or headed in that direction. You have a lot of room for improvement and you can see that you can modify most of your current behaviors without difficult adjustments. This book may actually help you avoid the progression to a serious illness lurking right around the corner.

(Note: This short quiz does not factor in the relationship of your genetics to your habits of health score. Go to www.habitsofhealth.net to take the full assessment.)

ARE YOUR DAILY CHOICES MOVING YOU TOWARD HEALTH OR DISEASE?

Here are two very important takeaways from the questionnaires:

- You now know where you are along the continuum of optimal health, non-sick, or sick. Most people think they are doing okay until they have a heart attack or stroke. If you are not optimally healthy, you are at risk.

- Second, you now understand the importance and influence of the simple decisions about what you eat, how you move, and how you think about and act on your health.

All these seemingly small choices are more powerful when combined and integrated than any medicines or medical miracles that we think we can rely on for help. Your decline along the continuum toward disease doesn't have to be inevitable. You can start to reverse the downward slope today by choosing to take an active role in your health. The first step is to understand that no one is going to do it for you. No doctor, friend, family member, or medical institution is going to change your path.

Ask yourself a few questions:

- What's my current mind-set regarding health? (Do I depend on my doctor for my health?)

- Do I take action to improve my health every day?

- Are my daily habits creating a vibrant, healthy, energetic life, or leading me to be tired and in decline?

These questions challenge the choices you've been making about your life. They challenge not just your mind-set, but the next choice you'll make about what you eat, how you move, and whether or not you'll smoke, drink, or take harmful drugs. When you have a mind-set of health, you put health in the center of each day. Part of that decision involves uncovering and dispelling any myths.

In my work as a physician, I have observed that one of the biggest myths people believe is that family history plays the biggest role in determining health. Genetics do play a role but not as big a role as daily habits and choices. People say, "I've got big bones," "Everyone in my family is heavy," or, "Everybody in my family dies young." Those are excuses or blind spots that prevent people from living the healthiest life they can. Approximately 30 percent of your health is determined by your genetics, and 70 percent is within your control by changing your choices and environment.

Even if several people in your family have suffered from heart disease, the fact still remains that 90 percent of cardiovascular disease is preventable.

Your lifestyle determines your heart health. Daily exercise (how much you move your body), nutrition (the foods you choose to eat), quality sleep, and how you handle stress are more important determining factors to how healthy your heart will be.

The small daily habits and choices you make, not one huge thing, change the state of your health. That's why there has never been any one medication, herb, or diet supplement that by itself has created long-term health. There is no magic bullet. You're the dominant force in your life, not your genetics, family history, or what other people are doing.

In my opinion, every medical professional should be principally concerned with helping people live in optimal health. My mission and focus is to move medicine to a different place, where it is truly a health-care rather than sick-care industry. In the next chapter, I explain why this is so important, not just for you but for the United States.

CHAPTER 3

Selling Sickness

America's health care system is
neither healthy, caring, nor a system.[1]
—Walter Cronkite

START THIS CHAPTER WITH A DISCLAIMER. I'm a physician and very proud of that fact. I'm also proud of the millions of physicians who have the goal to serve humankind at great personal sacrifice.

The U.S. medical delivery system is among the best in the world; its doctors are incredibly talented at helping sick people—someone who has been hit by a car or who needs open-heart surgery, for example. When I was in my residency at Cleveland Clinic, I was amazed how many famous people were attracted there. Nobility, diplomats, and stars from around the world came to have their heart operations performed at the Cleveland Clinic because we averaged over twenty open heart operations a day with amazing results. With that much practice, you can get really good. In today's medical world, if you need a coronary artery bypass or aortic valve replacement, you are in luck. But if you want to create radiant health in your life, you are asking the wrong industry for help.

SICK CARE DOES NOT
FOCUS ON HEALTH

The medical industry is focused on sick care, not health care. It focuses on making you better when you are sick, not keeping you well. My vision for all people is that they live to be one hundred years old, in great health and without disease. We should all spend our last years with a whole generation of centenarians whom we have known since birth. But the current reality is quite different. Far too many individuals spend their last decades and certainly their last year with progressively debilitating diseases that rob them of their vitality. Their days are filled with doctor visits, medications with bothersome side effects, and therapies that often inflict great pain and suffering.

The United States spends over $2.3 trillion a year on health care. One leading cause of the spending is the $500 billion pharmaceutical industry. The United States, with less than 5 percent of the world's population, makes up almost 50 percent of the global market for prescription medicines. Sick care is big business and has spawned suppliers that provide symptom abatement and disease management. But what about America's health?

Prescription medications are among the top causes of mortality in patients. The United States is ranked 37th in terms of health among the 191 members of the World Health Organization, and 72nd in terms of overall level of health.[2] The country has veered way off course in how it addresses caring for the health of its citizens. The focus of the health-care industry is on reacting to diagnosis and disease. It has spun into a multi-trillion dollar industry of sick care.

It wasn't always so. If we trace the development and focus of modern medicine to its origins, we can distinguish three key periods of advancement.

THE FIRST ERA OF MEDICINE

The first era began during the golden age of classical Greece. Hippocrates separated the discipline of medicine from religion, believing and arguing that disease was not a punishment inflicted by the gods but rather the product of environmental factors, diet, and living habits. His therapeutic approach was based on "the healing power of nature." According to this doctrine, the body contains the power to rebalance and heal within itself. Hippocrates, considered the father of Western medicine, preached "first do no harm," which is included in the oath I took over thirty years ago.

This first era of medicine accelerated in 1928 with the discovery of penicillin. With immunizations and improved public health, during the first half of the twentieth century, we were able to extend our lives by several years and even decades. The advent of antibiotics as magic bullets to stamp out infection in a sick person gave great hope that we could use advancing technology to eradicate many diseases.

THE SECOND ERA

In the second era of medicine, we declared war against chronic disease and set out to find cures for the next great threats to our health, such as heart disease, stroke, cancers, diabetes, and other diseases that diminish the quality and the length of life. We have made improvements in diagnostics and medical care, and have witnessed a significant decline in cigarette smoking. Some drugs, like cholesterol-lowering drugs, have helped in preventing people from dying of cardiovascular disease. However, in other areas, such as cancer, we have made little advancement.

Beyond extending life, we have done very little to prevent or reverse disease. The real advances have been a whole lot of technologies and pharmaceuticals that have driven up costs and put health care on the precipice of bankrupting the country. Why has this happened?

Our successes targeting bacteria with specific antibiotics have distracted us from discovering the important cause of disease. Why do we have disease? Is it a part of life, or can it be prevented? Magic bullets, antibiotics, antivirals, and vaccines are so successful because they target external, invading organisms. They are not attacking disease in our organs. (Vaccines stimulate the immune system by mimicking a foreign organism invading the body.) We assumed that disease, beyond infections, was also caused by something outside. But when we look at why we get diseases, it has everything to do with our inside world.

The focus of health care today is managing chronic disease through management of symptoms. The current medical community philosophy is that if we can diagnose and categorize a symptom or disease, we can treat it with a medication. The current thinking is that if we can do more diagnosis, we can find a more specific drug. Recently, the World Health Organization transitioned from 12,000 possible diseases in the International Classification of Diseases (ICD) ICD-9, the medical profession's organized system of coding all disease, to more than 150,000 possible diagnoses in ICD-10. They increased the categories over ten times. If you are a pharmaceutical company, this is good news. You can develop more specific medications to treat all these new labels.

In contrast, I am devoting all my energy to go in a different direction and focus on a different outcome. What if we focus on partnering with patients to give them what they really want?

THE THIRD ERA

In this new, third era of medicine, the challenge is for physicians to focus on what is in a patient's best interests, instead of more medicines or surgery. This is about patients living longer, healthier lives without disease or medication or frequent trips to the doctor. This partnership goes beyond using the current biomedical model approach to a patient, with its focus on treating organs, rather than people.

As I discussed in the previous chapter, metabolic syndrome is a lifestyle-induced cluster of metabolic derangements and symptoms that leads to diabetes, cardiovascular disease, and eventually death. It has an impact on several organs. The symptoms of high blood sugar, blood pressure, and high cholesterol are all warnings from your body that your fat cells are filled and your body is not processing carbohydrates well. So your choice is to:

- Take a bunch of expensive medicines and develop progressive disease that can affect your eyesight, extremities, heart, kidneys, and sex life.

  or

- Address it by eating healthier and adopting the habits of health. Hippocrates' idea that the body can heal itself is still valid today.

Going from your youthful state of health to succumbing to a diabetes-related heart attack may take decades. But if diabetes is diagnosed early and reversed, the heart attack could be prevented because you've helped your body heal itself. Or better yet, diabetes never occurs because you decide to change your daily choices now and make health a priority.

If I can encourage you to use the strategies, skills, and tools of the habits of health, you will be better informed when you go to your physician. You'll discover the real value of diagnostics, early detections, and checkups. This new mind-set will put you in a wonderful position to live a longer, healthier life.

Developing healthy habits is a subject I'm passionate about. After years as a physician in the traditional medical world, I've seen the devastation from unhealthy lifestyles. Despite ever-advancing technology, I knew we were losing the fight against the habits of disease. Yet, as I have mentioned before, my training was transformational in understanding that when the parts that make up the whole body are integrated, a patient's overall health is improved. Instead of focusing on one symptom or body part, you focus on everything—the causation, prevention, and intervention.

Guiding patients to create healthy new daily habits (and replace old ones) is the job of a physician concerned with helping people live in optimal health. It is about creating teachable moments. It's about a lifestyle of health and healthy choices, not a one-off quick fix.

Small daily habits and choices can change the state of your health. The power for health is in your hands, not your physician's.

You are your health's keeper.
And it really matters.
As you shall soon see!

> The . . . patient should be made to understand that he or she must take charge of his own life. Don't take your body to the doctor as if he were a repair shop.[3]
>
> **Quentin Regestein**

CHAPTER 4

Does Health Really Matter?

Man sacrifices his health in order to make money. Then he sacrifices money to recuperate his health. . . . He lives as if he is never going to die, and then dies having never really lived.

—Unknown

THE PURSUIT OF SUCCESS WITHOUT REGARD for the effect on our health is one of our greatest errors. It is as if someone sat us down at the beginning of our careers and whispered in our ears: "Be successful!"

Desiring more for yourself and your family is fine; making money is usually a good thing. But success, not health, becomes the center of our lives, which is why most people become unhealthy after a certain age. Most people strive each day to earn more, buy more, and achieve more. There is no direct correlation between success and the potential for fulfillment, joy, happiness, or emotional security.

But without your health, you really have nothing. My goal is to help you place health at the center of your life and success as an offshoot. With health as the hub, success, financial reward, happiness, travel, kids, and family can all exist as spokes of the wheel. You will enjoy everything much more if you're not sidelined with medications, medical bills, and doctor visits.

However, you cannot enjoy material things or the experiences with friends and family, if you are stressed about how to pay for them. You cannot have the best time with your kids or grandchildren if you are short of breath when you play with them.

If I could whisper in your ear right now I would say, *be optimally healthy*. There is a direct correlation between your sense of well-being and your mental and physical health. Let's think about what a healthy human looks like.

Visualize some young children playing all day in a swimming pool. Their laughter echoes across the water, and they jump in and out of the water and run to the diving board despite parental warnings to slow down. Their energy and noise levels are so high that their parents enforce rest periods just so they can catch their breaths. During those rest periods, the stressed-out adults can enter the water to cool down without worrying about being splashed. The adults may even move a few feet and stretch their arms across the water before once again retreating to lounge chairs to lie in the sun and escape the chaos of their crazy lives for a few hours. The children, on the other hand, go nonstop for several more hours until their bodies switch off. As the sunlight fades, parents struggle to their cars, carrying these fifty-pound dynamos, now inanimate objects deep in a restful sleep that the adults so desperately need but cannot seem to capture.

We have all experienced those same moments in our lives. We were all born into this world with energy and vitality. Then life and success and work got in the way. The responsibility of being adults changes our schedules, time, and priorities.

Now you get up early to go to work, take the kids to school, and get the chores done. You are tired, stressed out, and worn out, and have just enough energy to fall into bed at the end of the day. Tomorrow, you'll get up and do it all over again. Over and over, month after month, year after year, you pay the toll as this schedule saps your energy and erodes your health. Maybe you are already on medications, seeing doctors, and just barely surviving. Or maybe you're moving so fast that everything seems fine physically—for now. You may have even bought into the dogma that this pattern is inevitable and there is nothing you can do about it.

Nothing could be further from the truth. Every day, there are reminders to eat right and work out. Magazine covers scream at the checkout line. When a friend is diagnosed with cancer, you're reminded about your own health. You wonder about your friend's symptoms, the first pains he or she had. Each week, you're reminded that your current behaviors are either destructive or productive for your health. Each day, you make the choice to walk down the path of living habits of disease or health.

Now is the time to choose healthy habits and eliminate the habits of disease. The day in the life of a healthy child that I just described is one that I experienced with healthy adults just last year. I was playing water volleyball at a retreat in Punta Cana, with several coaches who have used the habits of health to go from surviving to thriving. I watched as this diverse population of previously overweight, obese, and unhealthy individuals played for several hours. Ranging in age from the mid-twenties to the mid-seventies, these adults were laughing, screaming, high-fiving, and just having fun. Their energy was high and nonstop. As the match extended from the best-out-of-five games to five out of seven, I had an epiphany that all things in terms of our health are possible. These barely surviving individuals had transformed into fun-loving, competitive, healthy kids again. These ordinary people were taking extraordinary care of their health.

It is possible for you as well.

In these introductory chapters, I have taken you through a process of self-discovery to give you the knowledge and understanding to prepare you for your journey. In chapter 1, I outlined the hostile obesegenic environment that surrounds you. In chapter 2, you found your current health status and the direction of your daily habits. In chapter 3, I discussed sick care's role and put you in charge of your health. In this chapter, we are beginning to explore the extreme contrast between excellent, vibrant optimal health and the survival mode that most people live in.

Let's look at your health in more detail to deepen your appreciation of how precious and amazing it really is.

WHY IS HEALTH SO IMPORTANT?

Your body has the inherent capacity to heal itself. When it is healthy, it can navigate through adversity, accidents, and stressful times, and come out on the other side in great shape.

Remember when you were a kid and fell, scraping your knees, or you broke a bone falling out of a tree. It might have been painful, but in only days, you were running and climbing again. A high school sporting event or team competition was stressful, but you had that extra burst of adrenaline and made it through it just fine. In college, a late-night party on Saturday might have almost done you in, but it didn't. Sunday morning, you suffered a pounding hangover, vowing "I will absolutely never drink again." Yet, by Monday morning, magically you were as good as new and even aced your exam.

My point is that the body has amazing recuperative abilities. It did then, and it does now, but it takes a little more time. And only if you've continued to create daily habits of health that propel you along the path of health for life. But when Saturday night drinking turns into a daily event or eating rich unhealthy food goes from an occasional celebration dinner to three meals a day, year after year, your body is in harm's way.

The same goes for stress, whether the daily stress of a nonfulfilling occupation, a difficult daily commute, or a disharmonious life at home. When you are stressed all the time, your body starts to lose its edge.

Hans Selye, a Hungarian endocrinologist, uncovered the deleterious effects of chronic stress on our bodies. His research revealed that an overstimulated autonomic nervous system leads to a plethora of long-term negative effects on health.[1] Hormonal changes, musculoskeletal imbalances, and suppression of the immune system can rapidly take you from a non-sick to a sick state. Stress is now directly implicated in the onset of many cancers, such as breast, esophageal, and prostate cancers. Stress can also produce or worsen diabetes, heart attack, stroke, and many of the diseases that lead to death. We are literally worrying ourselves to death.

People who are engaging in unhealthy behaviors frequently say to me (before they understand), "You have to die of something." True, but why hasten it? They believe that attitude gives them license to live fast and do whatever they want, so they continue to smoke, overeat, or drink too much, oblivious to the consequences. But as a physician, I can tell you that it matters in many ways. For twenty years, I took care of patients who insisted on continuing the high-risk habits of disease. Many preceded their predicted ultimate demise, when they "died of something," with many unnecessary years of sickness and a poor quality of life.

In the case of lifelong smokers, fewer than 10 percent actually get lung cancer. Of those that do, fewer than one in five survive more than five years of what is usually a very horrible death. But for those who are lucky enough to avoid the Big C, luck runs out. The result of years of inhaling unhealthy nicotine and smoke take a toll on their ability to breathe. Chronic obstructive pulmonary disease (COPD) is a horrible, progressive destruction of the lungs resulting in several years of gasping for air. In medicine, the symptom is called shortness of breath. This term does not accurately describe the condition. Imagine being a kid back in that swimming pool. Now visualize diving to the bottom of the deep end to pick up a coin. You have a feeling of angst as you pick up the coin and look at how far away the surface is. You feel as if your lungs will burst as you race back to the surface. Gasping for air, you take deep replenishing breaths, thinking you will never get enough air. Now imagine living every moment of the rest of your life with that feeling.

I have haunting memories of looking into the eyes of patients, seeing how scared they were, gasping to get enough air. Nothing is sadder for a physician than seeing people who no longer have any control over their health.

Some countries are realizing that health matters a lot and are doing something about it. A *New England Journal of Medicine* article discussed a ruling by the High Court of Australia on August 12, 2012, that upheld the constitutionality of tobacco laws.[2] The ruling directs all cigarette companies to cease selling their cigarettes in attractive, sexy packaging. Bright colors and macho or feminine labels can lure kids as well as adults to smoke and create an illusion that smoking is desirable. Australia is taking a vested interest in its citizens by helping them make a better choice. Now tobacco sellers must advertise with real photos showing graphic images of the health consequences of smoking. Mouth ulcers, lung tumors, and gangrenous limbs really aren't sexy.

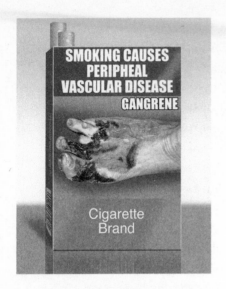

This photo is a duplicate of the actual cigarette packaging being mandated by the Australian government. It provides an ultimate reality check on what the habit of smoking does to the human body.

You may think that's not you because you don't smoke. But the end result from not exercising, or choosing poor-quality foods is the same. Obesity, a sedentary lifestyle, continuing to eat the wrong foods, and too much stress all lead to disease such as insulin resistance, diabetes, or inflammatory vascular disease. They are all part of the continuum as the body starts unraveling due to constant attacks by the habits of disease. Although America probably isn't ready for French fries packaged with graphic labels like the Australian cigarette cartons, it is ready for enhanced awareness of the health impact of our daily choices.

If patients overwhelm the medical delivery system by continued daily ingestion of unhealthy food, soon the U.S. government may be forced to follow Australia's precedent and put labels such as this on unhealthy food:

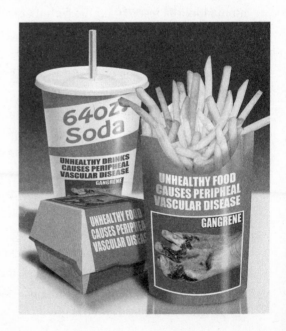

Another reason your health matters is the advancing ability to treat disease and prolong life. Great strides have been made in reducing death resulting from the habits of disease. Since 1950, death from cardiovascular disease has been reduced by approximately 65 percent.[3] What we have not done is help those same patients create health. So the burden of decreasing functionality and poor-quality lives remains, as most citizens are living longer, but unhealthy lives. See the correlation? We are prolonging life, but an *unhealthy* life.

Life expectancy is at an all-time high. That means you are probably going to have to live with the pain and discomfort that comes from an unhealthy lifestyle for a longer time. For perspective, think of the analogy of the American car. In the 1950s through the 1970s, the American auto industry dominated the market. Automakers built planned obsolescence into their vehicles. They would change the look every year, enticing customers to buy the latest, greatest car with the new tail fins. Those who could afford a new car didn't see the need to take good care of their current cars; they knew they would soon discard them. Most of those cars are no longer on the road.

At a medical conference in Cuba a few years ago, I was amazed to see that all the cars from the 1950s were still on the road there and in good condition. Because of the embargo, Cubans have not been able to get parts for their U.S. cars for almost sixty years. Yet, with loving care and proper maintenance, the cars are purring along in Havana, after more than half a century. We could learn some lessons from the Cubans about maintaining our bodies, because an embargo on resources to treat disease is looming.

The steps for becoming the dominant force in your health are not difficult. The steps also take less time than you might think. I understand that time is your most precious resource. You are pulled in many different directions and have no time to go to gyms consistently. Finding healthy foods can be a hassle, and often they aren't available. The kids wake you up at night, and caffeine seems to be the only fuel that gets you through the day.

My life is like yours. I am a father, a husband, a doctor, a writer. I'm traveling all the time. Like you, I'm living in the same obesegenic world you are. Are we thriving? Or just surviving? I know you can't imagine how you are going to find the time to get healthy. But I have figured it out and will help you do the same.

THE INCONVENIENCE OF DISEASE

As a doctor, I have seen a drastic shift in the allocation of free time as people head down the pathway to disease. The inconvenience of being tied to six or seven medications multiple times a day, as well as the cost and debilitating side effects, can rob your quality of life. For some, it may involve daily finger pricks and self-administered shots of insulin. Then there's inconvenience of monthly or weekly office visits with multiple specialists and their lengthy wait times. (So much for being irritated about a thirty-minute wait for pizza.) How about those inconvenient emergency room visits or lengthy hospitalizations? Or the inconvenience of wearing a CPAP mask to bed to prevent airway obstruction and snoring, while hoping your spouse is in the mood? (She won't be.) Or the inconvenience of your kidneys no longer functioning, so you have to go to a dialysis center instead of your bathroom to clear the toxins from your body?

You may already be dealing with some of these issues. If so, you most likely agree that disease is indeed inconvenient.

• • •

I am going to help you become as optimally healthy as possible, despite your current position on the health continuum. I am not trying to make you feel guilty or scare you into action. Those of you who are not far down the health continuum need to understand the insidious trajectory from non-sick to disease and why it should matter.

Next, let's investigate why a healthy lifestyle seems so difficult and why you may have struggled to achieve it.

CHAPTER 5

Why Does It Seem So Difficult?

The only way to keep your health
is to eat what you don't want, drink
what you don't like, and do what
you'd rather not.[1]

—Mark Twain

THE PURSUIT OF OPTIMAL HEALTH, in Mark Twain's opinion, appears to be an almost insurmountable task. It seems so hard and undesirable that it may be something you would rather not do. I do not disagree. From where you are now, it probably seems too difficult or even impossible.

I have presented compelling reasons why you are currently unhealthy or about to be and why you need to pay attention to your health. But, given your busy life, making sacrifices that are unsustainable makes no sense.

I agree. It's like insanity, doing the same thing over and over and expecting a different result. So let's start from a different perspective.

Say you are standing outside in a park and it starts raining. You are going to get wet. You can say you are going to stay dry, but that is not going to happen. No matter how hard you think, you cannot use willpower to avoid getting wet. What tools can help you stay dry?

Umbrella Great tool to protect you from direct rain, but if it's windy, you are going to get wet.

Raincoat Keeps you generally dry, but your head, neck, legs, and shoes are going to get wet.

Rain hat Your head will be dry, but later you will have to deal with hat hair.

Rubber boots Your feet will be dry, but the rain running off your body may drip in.

So, there are several tools that can help you stay dry. But each one alone cannot keep your whole body dry. (And practically, if you are equipped with all of the tools on a sunny day in anticipation of a squall, you have some bigger problems than just getting wet.)

So why do we think that dieting on occasion, taking vitamins, going to a doctor annually, or exercising are going to keep us healthy? Our obesegenic, unhealthy world is raining on us from the time we get up in the morning until we attempt to shut it all off and go to bed.

Recently, a friend of mine was at a neighborhood party. As she looked around the room, she noticed that every single woman in her fifties or sixties was slumped on a chair or couch. All were overweight. She observed that each one had a rounded belly and swollen ankles. She wondered what had happened to them. She'd known them for years. Each had been vibrant and pretty. But now, a decade later, they all had the same round shape. Was it a coincidence? She hadn't seen any of them working out or even walking in the neighborhood. She thought that years of overindulgence and a sedentary lifestyle had caught up with them.

Is this what will happen to you? You know the habits of disease are leading you toward poorer and poorer health, but you keep thinking, "I just do not have time for myself." Or, maybe you exercise at the gym, yet eat whatever you want because you think it's okay because you exercised. But one cancels out the other. That's not the path to health. Or you skip breakfast to reduce calories, eat a high-fat fast-food lunch, and rationalize incorrectly that since you didn't have time for breakfast, you will be all right. You tell yourself that you will make it to the gym on Wednesday, but you are wondering why you are a pound heavier on Saturday. Your spouse starts nagging you daily, and your treadmill with the heart monitor attached is just an expensive, convenient place to hang your coat.

Where do people go wrong? Here are some comments I've heard from people I've coached:

- My mom told me to eat everything on my plate as a kid; today I still struggle with wasting all that good food.

- I keep having these moments when I feel guilty and then I decide to get healthier.

- I have tried every technique to get healthy. Some of them work; some of them don't.

- Some techniques work for a while, but always seem to fail over time. I have been trying to get rid of this extra weight for years now.

- Like my parents, I guess I am destined to be obese my whole life.

- My father died of a heart attack at age fifty, so why should I bother?

You may have had some or all of those thoughts at some point. But now is the time for a change in mind-set. This journey is going to transform your thinking and add years to your life.

TEN INFLUENCERS

The following ten categories are important influencers in the way we all see life, live life, and participate in the creation of the habits that lead to longevity. We are going to explore, modify, and transform them.

Our current world. In chapter 1, I described our nutritionally polluted world. Add in a sedentary lifestyle, stress, information overload, and lack of time, the food industry, and even the influence of your friends.

Your new world. You are going to change the underlying structure of your world. To further the example of rain in the park and how an umbrella or hat might be helpful, imagine a building in the park that you could enter and stay dry. We are going to build such a structure. Although we cannot remove all threats, you will dramatically reduce your exposure as you are surrounded in a microenvironment of health.

Your design. Ten thousand years ago, the design of your body served you well. Everything humans ate was nutritionally dense and energy sparse. They picked and ate berries because calories were scarce, and their 40 billion fat cells gobbled up the extra calories for future use. In addition, humans worked very hard to procure food and foraged all day long. They went to sleep when the sun went down and the campfire went out.

Your current mind-set. I'm going to help you create a new mindfulness. Unless you are aware and focused, you will default to your previous programming. The first step is that you learn and become mindful of your surroundings. You will become more aware of everything, from picking your food choices in grocery stores and restaurants to your daily fitness decisions. You will get moving more, without the gym. You will develop the mind-set so you can discover your optimal health.

Your time. Time is one of your most valuable resources. We all thought that technology was going to create a more relaxed, shorter workweek. But the reality is that we are working over an hour more than people worked in 1950. And because both parents work, our children and chores consume the nonwork time. Life now includes more high-tech gadgets, a cleaning person, and two cars. It is time to concentrate on your needs, your health, and your body and mind.

Your choices. You need to prioritize your tasks, tools, a plan, and support. I will help you create the habits you need and add the necessary adjustments into your schedule to place you on the path to optimal health.

Problem-solving orientation. You are programmed to get up in the morning and react to whatever is in front of you. You have become really proficient at problem solving to keep it all together. Yet you are not getting closer to being healthier or saner. You're just putting out fires, instead of creating a new life.

Health orientation. You are going to learn to shift your focus toward what is most important to you. Your health should be at the top of the list.

Your current plan. If you have a plan, and many do not, it probably relies for the most part on dieting and/or exercise. You have probably tried all kinds of techniques to motivate yourself. Dieting comes in many different flavors and styles. How have they worked out? If you have been beating yourself up because your diet never lasts, you are not alone. Eighty-five percent of people who go on a diet have gained their weight back within two years.

Your new plan. I am going to help you address all the logistical and psychological aspects of your life. You are a unique individual. You will create your optimal health plan around your needs.

TIME TO RECALIBRATE

All the healthful things you have thought, envisioned, or actually done in the past are irrelevant. Now is the time to start with a blank slate. I'm going to help you shift the focus from external control to internal, intrinsic control. Simply put, you are in control. It doesn't matter if your spouse or friend continually nags you, because it has no long-lasting value and can actually be one reason you are not working on your health. It doesn't matter if you've had guilt, shame at being overweight, or other emotions that do not create meaningful change. You will abandon those old mind-sets, actions, or techniques to really focus on what you want.

Let's explore now what that new radiant health is going to look like.

CHAPTER 6

From Should to Would

A healthy outside starts from the inside.[1]

—Robert Urich

WHEN YOU REALIZE THAT YOU SHOULD MAKE health a priority and do something about it, you may look for a technique or system to help you change. Bookstores and infomercials are full of the latest techniques for motivating or helping you, and the more desperate you are, the more likely you will try the most unlikely solutions. Cookie diets, boot camps, deprivation therapy, pineapple diets—the list is endless. One of my favorite quick fixes advertised is the belt with electrodes that you wrap around your waist to "melt the fat away." Really? Does anyone think that works? This purchase would be an emotional one. It would make more sense to put the belt on your forehead for shock therapy and ask, "What was I thinking?"

Should

CORE MEANING: modal verb indicating that something is the right thing for somebody to do; **used** to advise somebody to do something.

In order to make health a priority, you've got to have a deep, authentic, personal desire to change and create health. That desire only occurs when you've realized that your health really is that important. This decision affects the rest of your life.

Would

CORE MEANING: used to express the sense of "will." To want, to do it because it is your choice.

ARE YOU READY TO TAKE RESPONSIBILITY FOR MANAGING YOURSELF?

I can't motivate you to change, and there are no techniques that can. I know that statement may contradict anything you've heard in the past about weight loss or health. But what I've learned after working with thousands of individuals and families is that it's all about *you*. In the end, the decision is yours.

Success comes when you are really ready to change. I can help educate you about the importance of your health. I can explain how to overcome the barriers that have made getting healthy a struggle, and I also can guide you through some of the psychological hurdles you may have had with dieting, triggers, and emotional eating. But the one-thousand-pound elephant in the room isn't me, your family, what you ought to do, or a lack of time. It's your own desire to live a healthy life.

This book is about offering you a new approach to managing your life. It's about getting real with yourself and having a partner who cares about your success. I've helped thousands of people go from merely surviving to thriving in long-term, radiant health. During the journey, I've learned the powerful truth that success boils down to intrinsic motivation. Intrinsic motivation comes from within.

As we make our way through life, two very different forces determine our choices and behaviors. The first force is doing things because we want to. The excitement and initiative comes from within. We do them because we are interested and they matter to us. The second force is control from outside. We do things because we feel pressured to do them. This type of behavior has become very prevalent today. We may comply because someone tells us to act a certain way or exerts authority over us. Or the opposite is true. Sometimes when we feel controlled or pressured to do something, we do the reverse, just because it feels better or more natural to push back. You may have someone nagging you to lose weight or stop eating those unhealthy snacks (and you know they are right), but you just keep doing it. That's because no one can tell you to do what you aren't ready to do.

It all comes back to intrinsic desire. So, ask yourself—are you ready to make your health a priority?

MAKE ONE SMALL CHANGE

You now know that it's a lot easier to make small, incremental changes in your daily habits and choices than to be riddled with inconvenience of disease for the rest of your life. If you're really ready to make your health a priority—and I think you are—you don't have to make insurmountable changes. You have everything you need. You don't have to join an expensive gym and buy workout gear and costly supplements. You don't need to plan an elaborate schedule that interrupts your life, yet may be short-lived. The tools I'm giving you revolve around making health the center of your life, not an unrealistic external goal, action, or item to fit into your schedule. The habits I'm encouraging you to develop will fit into your life naturally each day.

There's nothing that can make up for the incredible sense of well-being you have when you are healthy. No matter how much money you have made, fame you have won, or possessions you have accumulated, once your health has vanished, all those material things won't matter.

If you've ever been around someone who had it all and then suddenly got sick, you know what I'm talking about. Sickness can come on like a thief in the night, robbing them of time, plans, vacations, and dreams. I know from looking in the eyes of my critically ill patients on their deathbeds that the size of their portfolios or their fast sports cars did not matter. None of it mattered when they were fighting for life.

The health assessment you did in chapter 2 is a reality check. It gives you the cold truth about your current and future levels of health. It's aligned with your current behavior. Which path will you choose? The positive path to health or the negative path to disease?

IT'S YOUR CHOICE

You now understand that no amount of technology can rescue you from the impact of habits that detract from health. If you have adopted a pattern of negative daily habits, you've placed yourself on the trajectory from non-sick to eventual sickness. This habit of disease path is very difficult to reverse if you are not decisive about changing it. Each day, the way you eat, move, sleep, and handle stress is leading you either toward health or away from it. The habits that lead to disease are draining your life account. It may not be detectable at first, but eventually those habits add up to illness or, even worse, a poor health diagnosis. Or, you can put yourself on the path to healthy habits by making choices that enhance your health.

It's that simple.

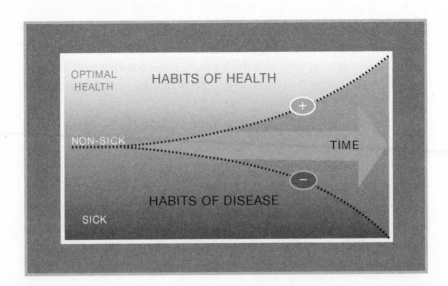

By now, you should be screaming, "There's no other choice! Get on the path to health!"

But just because you know you should, doesn't mean you will. If you're not ready, nothing will happen. If you are ready to get healthy—and reaching optimal health is a priority—let's walk this road together. If you are feeling overwhelmed or just not sure, ask yourself the following questions:

- Is there anything about my life and habits that could have a negative impact on my health or shorten my life span?

- Does my health matter enough to me now so I am ready to make health a priority?

Imagine what it would be like to live in vitality, to the age of a hundred. It's possible. More than five hundred thousand centenarians do it today. Can you become one of them? If you adopt healthy habits to reverse the effects of aging, damage, and habits of disease, you can.

Living a longer, healthier life is possible. I can help you change your trajectory and put you on that path to discover your optimal health. But I cannot make you want to do it. If you're not sure, take some more time to decide. I will leave you with something that no author, physician, wellness guru, or health expert has ever told you before. *If you are not really ready to change, don't bother to start, because the odds are drastically against you.* Why? Because meaningful change comes only when people feel that now is the time to change. When they feel pressured, they might comply for a while, but are not likely to maintain the change.

Once again, there is a reason why 85 percent of people who go on diets to lose weight gain it back within two years.[2] They weren't focused on creating optimal health. They were only focused on solving a problem they were running away from. See the difference? *What I'm proposing is to create, generate, and live in optimal health.*

The rest of the book is about integrating optimal health into your life. If you are ready to proceed, I am waiting to guide you on your journey.

CHAPTER 7

Your Health Guide and Compass

Motivation is what gets you started.
Habit is what keeps you going.[1]

—Jim Rohn

Y OU KNOW WHAT I LOVE ABOUT MY LIFE?
I can get up every morning and do something I'm passionate about. Each day, I'm living my dream. I make a difference in people's lives once they've decided they want to change. I know if someone really desires health and wants to live a longer, healthier life, I can help them.

So now that you have raised your hand, you are one of those people. You are my newest partner. So let's go to work.

STEP ONE:
UNDERSTAND MY ROLE AS YOUR COACH

The remainder of the book will explain your specific steps to create sustainable health in your life. I am going to ask you to give me permission to coach and guide you.

Traditionally, your doctor is an authoritarian figure who dispenses advice, scare tactics, and medicines. You sheepishly comply (at least for a while) or, if the doctor's instructions are too tough a pill to swallow, you may reject them by being noncompliant.

As your guide and coach, I am not that doctor. Instead, I'm your partner. I'm here to encourage you and offer my experience to help you rationalize through education why you want to take these steps. When I ask you to write something down or create a visual board, please do it for yourself (not me). There are many studies that support both the reinforcement and enhancement of success by writing down thoughts. Repetition deepens understanding and creates new wiring in the brain.

STEP TWO:
FIND YOUR *WHY*

The most critical first step is to understand *why* you want to get healthy. A clear understanding of what is motivating you and why is the foundation on which we build long-term, sustainable health. It's the first of many differences between this, other yo-yo diets, activity plans, or neat tips and techniques that you may use for a while and then discard. As I mentioned previously, optimal health is different for each of us.

So start with your *why*.

Why do you want to change your health? I want to make sure you clearly understand where you are right now. I will ask questions so you can focus, but in general, why does it matter?

How motivated are you to get healthy, on a scale of one (lowest) to ten (highest)? If your motivation level is currently *lower than a seven*, you are not ready and should either:

- Go back to the beginning of the book and start over.

- Put the book down and come back when you are ready.

Here are a series of questions that will help you understand your *why* and help you visualize your future health:

Why did you initially start reading this book? Why were you initially drawn to it? The key element here is to realize that you are reading this book because you deeply want to, not because your friends, your family, or your doctor insisted you do something. *You* are ready to improve the quality of your life.

Why are you reading this book now? I hope you are continuing to read because I have awakened your desire for health and you are anxious to get going.

The following emotions don't help you make sustainable change:

- Being ashamed at the way you look if you are struggling with your weight.

- Guilt if you have issues with alcohol and feel you are bad because you have been drinking a lot.

Motivations driven by emotions are not sustainable.

Why does your health really matter to you? For example, someone who needs to lose thirty pounds because she has difficulty moving due to excessive weight has sustainable motivation. A real reason to change for someone who is dealing with excessive alcohol use would be that he is tired of waking up with dulled senses or a hangover.

What are you most excited about accomplishing? Here is where visualization of the *desired outcome* of optimal health will involve you and *endorse* the action necessary to make meaningful change.

How do you see the creation of sustainable health changing your life? Visualizing how this will change your daily activities in both work and leisure has a strong impact. For example, you would be able to travel like a normal passenger on planes, if you now need an extension on the seat belt (which is a limiting outcome of bad habits), or you would be able to play with your grandchildren, if now you can't because you get short of breath. Both are very worthy and desirable outcomes.

How will this plan affect your health immediately? The immediate impact on your health is important to visualize. I have mentored thousands of people who have lost over a hundred pounds. They are now jumping out of airplanes, sailing, competing in marathons, and doing other activities they could not have dreamed possible a few years ago. For them, getting a good night's sleep or getting their tight rings off their fingers was the great first change.

How will this plan affect your health in a year? After a year of living the habits of health, you may experience significant physiologic rejuvenation. Think about the potential to reduce or eliminate medications, CPAP masks, walkers, and so on (I can make no guarantees, of course).

How will this plan affect your health in five years? My plan is designed to create long-term, sustainable health changes by putting you on a path and giving you the daily, sustainable choices that build your health. People I coached ten years ago are now truly thriving in all aspects of their lives.

Are you worried if you can really maintain the plan? Of course, you will have doubts. Reaching and maintaining optimal health evades over 95 percent of the population. Temporary remedies and techniques, exercise equipment, and diets do not create health. A strong *why* for the right reasons, combined with a specific plan to build skills, strategies, and support, does. Remember, you don't have to be perfect; you just have to get better over time.

What are you most worried about giving up? The things you will change will actually enhance the quality of your life. Your relationships will become stronger, your sense of taste will improve, as well as your overall well-being, to name just a few. Your whole life will be better when you have increased energy and vitality and a more youthful appearance.

STEP THREE:
LIST YOUR HEALTH OUTCOMES

I hope you wrote down your thoughts as I suggested at the beginning of this chapter and took time to answer my questions. Now I would like you to write down all your desired outcomes for your health, as we prepare for your journey. Summarize what you desire as you become as optimally healthy as you can and what that would look like. Make sure you list things you want to bring into your life instead of things you want to get away from.

Here are some guidelines and suggestions, which will help you move toward optimal health:

FOUNDATIONS OF OPTIMAL HEALTH

- Healthy eating, including vitanutrients (the vitamins, minerals, and trace elements required to optimize our bodies)
- Healthy weight and normal waist size
- Active lifestyle including walking program, weight resistance training, flexibility, agility
- Recuperative sleep
- Relaxation
- Healthy environment (clear, clean fishbowl)
- State of well-being
- System of healthy community and support

A wonderful way to crystallize your thoughts is to create a visual record by making an *optimal health story board*. On a large piece of heavy paper or cardboard, glue a series of pictures that represent your desired outcome in several key areas of health. Use some magazines with color photographs that you can cut out for a visual representation of your optimal health. I have made an optimal health board for years; it's on my desk to remind me of my constant focus on creating my best health.

Over the years, many patients and clients have told me how their visualizations have become reality. One fifty-year-old, a very overweight woman, put a picture of a woman skydiving, which had always been her childhood dream, on her health board. Growing up, she never had the resources to realize her dream. Unfortunately, as she became a successful businesswoman, she traded her health for success. Although financially able, she had gained so much weight that she was not physically able to skydive. Two years after creating her optimal health board and making many healthy choices, she skydived at the same location where the picture was taken.

The optimal health story board works, but it is not magic. Do step three. Right now. If you think you don't need to, I would strongly suggest you reconsider. As corny as the task may seem, understand there is a deep connection between pictures and our thought process. Those Corona beach commercials with the aqua water sell a lot of marginal-tasting beer!

STEP FOUR:
USE YOUR HEALTH COMPASS

Now that you have written down your health outcomes and created your optimal health story board, you need to make choices as part of your daily habits of health. When you are clear about what you want and why it is important to you, it becomes a priority. You start organizing your choices around it. It's a powerful motivator.

On May 25, 1961, President John F. Kennedy announced before a special joint session of Congress the dramatic and ambitious goal of sending an American safely to the moon before the end of the decade. This dramatic initiative created a powerful vision that focused the United States on mobilizing and integrating resources to put an American on the moon. Supercomputers, astrophysics, and some of the most brilliant minds in the world achieved this goal on July 20, 1969, when Apollo 11 commander Neil Armstrong stepped off the lunar module's ladder onto the moon's surface.

Vision guided us to achieve our desired outcome. But the guidance system made it possible. How much of the time was Apollo 11 actually on course? Two percent! Ninety-eight percent of the time, the spacecraft was actually off course. How could there have been that many mistakes, yet the module landed on the moon? Because the gyroscope, a fascinating piece of equipment, pointed to the moon, no matter which way the spacecraft was actually positioned. With the moon as the destination, the compass heading was continually adjusted by a microprocessor to keep the craft moving toward its destination.

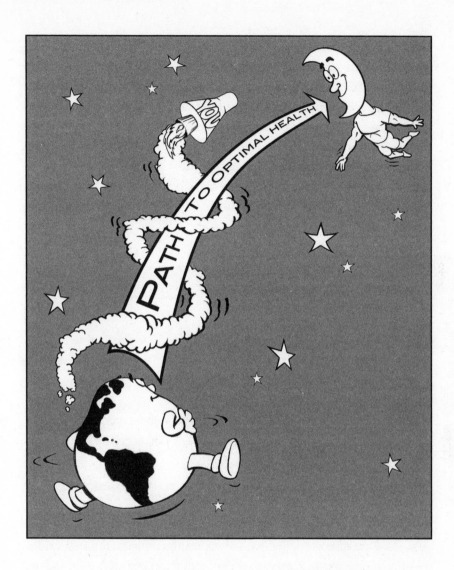

Your vision of optimal health as your desired outcome is a powerful gyroscope that can keep you on course as you continue to move toward living a longer, healthier life. It becomes your North Star. But you have to know where you are going if you're going to get there.

However, just like the spacecraft, you are going to get off course. In the past, when you were trying to be perfect, you probably blew your diet or started smoking again. This plan is not about being perfect. Once you are clear about your choices, it is simply about going into action, evaluating your progress, making the necessary corrections, and then going back into action. You do not beat yourself up if you make a mistake or make an unhealthy choice. What if Edison had quit after testing only ten filaments? Or Lincoln had quit after he lost his first political race? Instead, you will evaluate your actions and make the necessary adjustments. You cannot let an occasional backslide affect your overall goal, which is to deliver long-term, radiant health.

After you finish your optimal health story board, you have a picture of why you are making those healthy choices. Where are you going to display it?

SUGGESTIONS:

- Workspace
- Refrigerator
- Door to your garage
- Over your TV screen
- Your bathroom mirror
- On your smartphone (Take a picture of your health board with your smartphone so you can carry it around with you and look at it when tempted by the habits of disease.)

You are now equipped with your health compass, the first critical piece of equipment to keep you on course during your journey. It's a great way to stay on track as you develop the skills to learn the habits of health. As a fundamental choice, optimal health will help you make the right decisions. Over time, the healthy choices will become second nature, but for now use your compass daily to guide your choices.

Focusing on what you want is a powerful motivator, even when the going gets tough. Emotions can cause us to act initially, but over time, they usually let us down. They certainly interfere with our ability to continuously improve our health, as we shall see in the next step.

STEP FIVE:
AVOID THE EMOTIONAL TRAPS

Humans experience an array of emotions surrounding five basic feelings: happiness, sadness, anger, fear, and shame. These emotions can be based on a normal response to a real situation. If you went to a funeral, for instance, appropriately you would feel sad. If someone dents your car, you feel angry. But deep feelings of negativity tend to get us to do things to stop the feeling. You may be obese and hate the way you look, so you feel awful.

Your good-intentioned doctor tells you if you do not control your diabetes, you will go blind. Emotional turmoil builds in you until you decide to do something about it. Your emotions have motivated you to change. Or feelings of fear or embarrassment may cause you to act, but they are short-lived. For instance, what if you go to a holiday party and a button flies off your shirt and hits a guest. You may be so ashamed and embarrassed that you decide to go on a diet. You pick a four-hundred-calorie a day diet that causes you to lose weight (unfortunately, it is using muscle as your energy source, but more on that later). When you get on the scale, you're ten pounds lighter, so you put on that same shirt and it fits. You feel so good, you go out and celebrate and have a big, juicy cheeseburger and fries. You are off your diet.

Now you gain weight and enter the yo-yo dieting cycle. This kind of motivation is not going to help you reach and sustain optimal health. So before you go out into the unhealthy world with your new health compass, make sure you are setting your gyroscope to the outcomes you really want and are not running away from some situation or problem. Intrinsic motivation, a deep, powerful desire, can catalyze sustainable change. Please answer the following questions:

If you could choose optimal health, would you make that choice? This is a trick question because all of us would choose optimal health if we could. I am not asking if you think you can, but if you would actually choose it. Our intentions are one thing. Our actions are another.

Is your desire for optimal health a seven-plus on a scale of one to ten? Are you now ready to learn what it will take to achieve optimal health? If your desire to change your health is seven or above and you are coachable and teachable, you have the right mind-set to discover your optimal health and the right health orientation.

Are you are trying to solve something by starting this program? As long as you are not trying to start this program to get rid of bad feelings or guilt, but because you are primarily focused on improving your health, you will be all right. Problem solving does not create anything, but just gets rid of something you do not want. In terms of your health, focusing on health can create optimal health. Focusing on disease will not lead you to health.

This chapter has been about learning how we are going to work together as partners. You have now learned exactly why you're focused on reaching your optimal state of health and sustaining it for the long term. You now have a clear vision and visual image of what that looks like. You also recognize that some emotional feelings have the potential to get in the way. You finally understand that as long as you focus on creating radiant health, you have a strong tracking mechanism to keep you on a course to optimal health. Next I discuss all the amazing ways to propel you toward a healthier you.

CHAPTER 8

Your Health Is All about the Little Things

As long as we are persistent in our pursuit of our deepest destiny, we will continue to grow. We cannot choose the day or time when we will fully bloom. It happens in its own time.[1]

—Denis Waitley

THE STARTLING TRUTH IS THAT 95 PERCENT of all humans are either failing or falling short of mastering their choices. So their choices either serve them or destroy them. How can that be? This occurs because the majority of our actions do not give us immediate feedback on their importance and in which direction they point us. So we are left with no immediate feedback. We make the choices that bring us instant gratification. We disassociate the cause-and-effect of our actions.

That fried calamari, the bread and butter, letting the dog out rather than walking him—with each choice, there's no detectable difference today or tomorrow. But over time, from the same decisions, day in and day out, we end up in the emergency room with chest pain or worse.

So if you look at the illustration below, you can see that the small, insignificant, positive things do very little *immediately* to have an impact on your trajectory toward better health. According to the graph, only

5 percent of the population makes consistent choices to maintain optimal health throughout life. Yet the choices are not difficult if we have the knowledge, a plan, and a desire to change. And note that once you make a decision to focus on healthy choices, in a matter of a month or so you will be well on your way to optimal health.

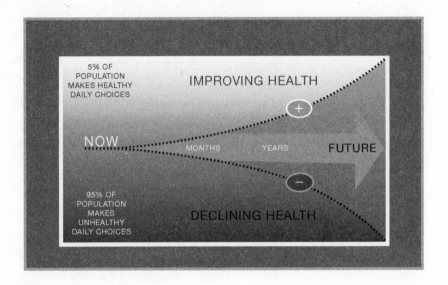

Note: This graph shows healthy (+) and unhealthy (−) choices, meaning that although we all do some things that are good for us, 95 percent of us are headed toward a non-sick state and, eventually, disease, because the summation of our unhealthy daily choices outweighs our healthy choices. But choices do make a difference sooner than later. They don't change you overnight, but they do change you. What the future holds for us as a civilization is hard to predict. What the future holds for you is determined by you.

I'm going to guide you to a new orientation, a new environment, and a series of continuous improvements in your daily choices. I will also ask you to reset your expectations so they are different from how you live your daily life now. In America, we demand instant gratification. You flip the light switch, and the light goes on. You go to the drive-through and expect the nutritionally polluted food delivered quickly. If the little old lady in front of you at airport security is struggling with all the procedures and moving slowly, you might get irritated. You want to move fast.

But this plan is about sustainability versus instant breakthrough. Discovering your optimal health involves taking a direct approach. It means putting into play 24/7 everything you do, every day, for the rest of your life. Its path involves being intentional about your food choices, your hundreds of daily movements, and the time and structure when you sleep. It involves how you handle yourself with your family and work associates. You are now going to take a thousand, small, insignificant, everyday actions and repurpose them to serve you.

In the last chapter, we established the first step to being as healthy as you can be. You now have a vision of what that will look like. In the chapters that follow, you will increase your understanding and shift your focus from knowing what to do to actually living the optimally healthy life. As Denis Waitley implies at the opening of this chapter, I cannot tell you how long it will take. I cannot guarantee you will get there. The odds are against you. So how do I keep you from getting impatient and giving up? How do I keep you from joining the gym in January and quitting by April? What can I do to prevent you from going on a diet and sticking to it for a couple of months, only to regain your weight? How can you avoid stopping cigarette smoking, only to revert to another habit of disease?

I am going to help you focus on what is most important and then make a lot of small adjustments in your daily activities. I want to teach you to be more mindful and not to look for the home runs, but to seek the walks and hits that allow you to create long-term health. It's not about taking the fun out of life. Optimally healthy people may eat lobster with butter or even have ice cream, but they don't do it every day.

Take a moment now to think about your actions in these situations and answer yes or no:

5 weeks in

	YES	NO
Eat breakfast every morning	+	–
Have small healthy meals	+	–
Eat pasta and rice	–	+
Eat fish 3 times a week	+	–
Take a 5-minute nap	+	–
Take an afternoon nap	–	+
Keep a routine	+	–
Drink 8 glasses of water per day	+	–
Your friends are overweight	–	+
Juice and blend your vegetables/whole	–	+
Wear clothes with an elastic waistband	–	+
Go for an intentional walk most days	+	–
Drink diet sodas every day	–	+
Spend time to meditate	+	–
Spend time with friends	+	–
Sit more than 5 hours a day	–	+

This is a small sampling of a bunch of some small little choices we make every day in our lives. Every one of them is easily done or not done. I know you are doing some of them right. Yet how many negatives do you have?

Look at them again and ask yourself if you could make the other opposite choice.

If the choice allowed you to improve your health in some small way, could you adopt it?

I know you can!

And you know you can.

It begins when you become aware of the many decisions that have an impact on your health and the trajectory of your life, you begin on the path to optimal health. And that requires you to be mindful, and in position to make good choices. For it has been said: First we make our choices; then our choices make us.

In the next chapter, we will begin on the first steps to choosing health as a priority.

CHAPTER 9

First Steps: Your Choice of Health as a Priority

Life expectancy would grow by leaps and bounds if green vegetables smelled as good as bacon.[1]

—Doug Larson

IF ONLY OUR CHOICES TO CREATE HEALTH could be easy. Yet mastering the discipline of making good choices is possible. Choices mean everything. Choice determines life or death, strength or mediocrity, career path or unemployment, strong relationships or shallow ones, healthy bodies or diseased ones. The choices we make determine how high we rise and how far we can go. If you wanted to be a world-class pianist, what would you do every day? *Practice.* Even if you came home from work so tired you just wanted to sit on the couch, you would go sit on the piano bench instead and practice. The primary choice, which is more important, guides you to do the secondary actions that support the primary choice. This fundamental principle is key to mastering your health. It is about saying no when you would rather say yes or saying yes when you would rather say no.

COVERING YOUR HEALTH BASICS

In this chapter, we will drill down on the choices that make all the difference. At the end of the chapter, I give you several things you can do right now to secure and protect your health. You may already be doing some of them, but you want to remove much of the chance for harm from your life now so the new optimally healthy you is well protected from external harm. I will also explain the cumulative impact of small, insignificant choices. The most important part of the habits of health and the ability to improve your health is not the knowledge *but the actual doing.* Most people think that having to focus on health is something that is not fun or easy to do. I disagree. Your health is a priority. You have made a decision to create health and you have a good idea what that looks like. Go back to chapter 2 and review your notes of where you currently are on the health continuum. *Please do it for you now.*

Study for a moment the contrast between your current health and choices and the new vision and desire you have for optimal health. What are you sensing? The discrepancy between what you want for your health and where your health currently is creates a dynamic state, which allows you to be energized to move toward optimal health.

Robert Fritz, author of the international best-seller, *The Path of Least Resistance*, has explored the relationship between vision and current reality as an important engine for creating meaningful change, called "structural dynamics." The tension caused by this discrepancy is structural; when you visualize the current and desired state simultaneously, it helps you focus on all the choices necessary to move forward. In the case of your health, it will become much easier to make the choices that support what is most important to you.

Fritz, who is a colleague, mentor, close friend, and a master of the creative process, talks about such choices as hierarchal. The more important choices dictate our motivation, and the secondary choices are things that we may not want to do, but because they are important for securing the desired outcome, we choose them anyway. Or we choose not to do what we would like to do because it moves us forward. I have adopted Fritz's important work into my optimal health coaching because it reinforces the forces in play in creating meaningful change. When we are intrinsically motivated and the originators of our actions, we can move forward toward our desired outcomes. This becomes a generative movement to resolve the discrepancy between our current health and our desire and motivation for optimal health.

THE HEALTH ORIENTATION

You can only get what you focus on. And you can focus on anything you want. If you decided to be a triathlete, you'd have a new bike, shoes, and spandex shorts. You'd buy running shoes and a swimsuit. And you'd be spending time running, biking, and swimming.

Once you have shifted your focus you will see right in front of you all the things that relate to that new focus. If you buy yourself a brand-new red convertible, within a few days you are driving around asking, where did all these red convertibles in your neighborhood come from? When we make something a priority and focus, we become aware of many things that were always right there in front of us but were previously unimportant to us.

Now that you have made health a priority and you know where you are, you will start making decisions that move you toward that goal.

You will now be aware of all the healthy choices you can make to move you toward your health goals. You will now look at the escalator and take the stairs.

You will see the bread on the table and ask the waiter to remove it.

There are hundreds of small decisions that you will make because they are now areas of focus and have become important to you in supporting your priority for health. You are the dominant force. You are the CEO of your health; you make the decisions that support living a longer, healthier life. You are no longer feeling that you are deprived when you do not eat the jelly doughnut or refuse a second helping of mom's pecan pie. You now make your choices based on what is most important to you. You will find many ways to eat healthier, move your body more, sleep better, and reduce your stress.

I observe with patients and clients that with this new orientation toward health, they find all kinds of innovative ways to make more positive decisions that are easier and more enjoyable than many of their old, unhealthier choices. And because the new choices support their fundamental choice for reaching their optimal state, their confidence and competence grow as well.

Another key area in helping you make more optimal health-directed choices and build your new Habits of Health is an increase in your mindfulness.

HEALTH MINDFULNESS

Another key to making more choices directed toward optimal health and building your new habits of health is to increase your mindfulness. Mindfulness is the ability to bring one's complete attention to the present experience, on a moment-to-moment basis. Most of us can make some improvements in this area. If you are not so sure mindfulness is a skill you need to hone, the next time someone at work is talking to you, ask yourself how many times you have drifted somewhere else.

I believe our technology has disconnected us from ourselves. As kids, we used to go out and spend the whole day in the woods alone or with friends. We would be very aware of our surroundings and negotiate our environment and relationships without distractions. We knew when we were hungry; we would pay attention and learn to open our hearts and cultivate kindness to each other. That has been lost in our disconnected, electronic world.

Now we go all day without regard for our body's needs or our colleagues' needs. We get upset for having bad thoughts or blame ourselves for slipping on our diets. We run to the habits of disease to make us feel better. Instead of heading out for a jog when we are stressed, we head for some sort of food or drink to relieve the stress.

When we are stressed, we activate our emotional brain and the limbic areas that lead us to reactive behavior. How does mindfulness relate to our choices (and the potential for developing healthy habits or unhealthy ones)? As humans, we are wired to experience sensations first through the emotional area of our brains called the limbic system. The signals then go to the prefrontal cortex where they stimulate a logical rational response.

This worked really well ten thousand years ago because if real danger were close, people would run and live rather than think and die. Even a hundred years ago, people were much more mindful of their surroundings and of others, and connected in stillness. People would sit in their living rooms at night and talk.

Today, we are so connected and distracted by other things that we have become much less mindful of our surroundings. Our faces are continually glued to iPads or iPhones from the moment we wake to the moment we fall asleep. Because of a lack of awareness or mindfulness, we are always in a reactive mode, tethered to our electronic leashes. This reactive state, charged with emotion, sabotages all our great intentions and can be a formidable adversary to creating optimal health.

Less than a third of us are even aware of these emotions, which if not managed correctly lead to unhealthy behaviors. So manage your emotions by first being aware or mindful. This critical first step is the undercurrent to everything you do. From this point on, you are going to become a mindful being, aware of your triggers and emotions. This allows you to understand and even direct your body chemistry, physiology, and action.

For instance, one woman finally realized that each day at precisely the same time—2 p.m.—she began feeling low. It was an emotional feeling she couldn't describe, but it was a lowering of satisfaction, energy, and happiness. To combat this low or depressed feeling, she would drink an alcoholic beverage. Or she would eat some chocolate or something sugary and instantly feel better. Her physiology changed from the habit, and her habits changed from the emotion or feeling inside her. It was a cycle. This went on for three years until she gained weight, was held hostage to the 2 p.m. blues, and then finally realized what was happening.

What emotions trigger you to make bad choices? If you can become aware of these emotions, it will give you a better chance of managing them in a healthy way. Managing the cycle and eliminating the things that don't serve you well is the new way of operating.

Before we start building all the small, incremental changes in your daily choices to help your body create its best possible health, let's talk about some of the choices that you should have already implemented. Copy this list and tape it to your refrigerator for others in your household to see.

MAKE THESE CHOICES RIGHT NOW:

- Eliminate all tobacco products now. (Remember the picture of the gangrenous foot on the Australian cigarette package?)
- Eliminate all recreational drugs.
- Wear your seat belt in your car and in taxis and limos.
- Buy a car with front and side airbags.
- Drive the speed limit; do not use a handheld phone.
- Be mindful of your surroundings all the time.
- Limit your intake of alcoholic beverages to fewer than two drinks a day.
- Never drink alcohol when driving or operating machinery.
- Switch to red wine if you do drink.
- Avoid situations that put you at risk for contracting sexually transmitted diseases.
- Avoid sunburn.
- Do not exercise on roads used by motor vehicles, if possible.

You may read that list and scoff at the simplicity of it. That means you don't yet understand that you can develop healthy habits and yet not have to avoid life. I love to sail and do what some people would consider extreme, such as racing my sailboat fifteen hundred miles across the ocean. We leave in November and sail from Hampton, Virginia, to Tortola in the British Virgin Islands. I prepare and skipper the boat, and my wife Lori and some close friends set out on an intense adventure. When you are eight hundred miles out in the middle of the ocean in a fifty-four-foot sailboat, you are very mindful of how self-reliant you are and the risks involved. Yet we are well prepared and equipped and have an amazing sailboat. I cannot describe how breathtaking the ocean is as the sunrise heralds a new day at sea. It is one of the times when I feel the most alive.

Yet, every day, when I get in my car, I reach over and fasten my seat belt because it is a habit of health. I want to stay alive! Seat belts save over two hundred thousand lives a year. This seemingly mundane habit can protect you and those you care about.

Healthy choices are not about avoiding life, eliminating fun things, or being a stick-in-the-mud. Live your life! Hike mountains, plan a trip to an exotic destination, jump out of a plane (with a parachute) if you want to. But every day, be sure you are making the positive, healthy choices that will lead to a stronger foundation for your life. The simple choices above, like limiting alcohol intake and not texting and driving, are far more critical decisions than determining if you're going to jump out of a plane once in your life.

> A risk-free life is far from a healthy life.[2]
>
> **Deepak Chopra**

Next are some ways to lay a foundation for a healthy life and ensure that you are making the right choices.

ANNUAL VISIT WITH YOUR DOCTOR

With my help, you now have a partner to help guide you toward optimal health. The next time you are at your doctor's office, tell him you are now focused on your health as a priority. You are adopting a health orientation and the habits of health that support living a longer, healthier life.

Since a great deal of medicine still depends on observation and interpretation, tell your doctor anything unusual you are experiencing. This is where mindfulness is important. You should discuss any new pains, symptoms, or change in your body's functions or patterns with your physician. You are with yourself 24/7 and have a much better vantage point of anything that has changed since your last visit.

Ask your doctor how he or she is staying current with the rapid technological advances and research. This won't be a popular question, so maybe you can research this a bit on your own with his staff or via the Internet. Remember, though, that you're in control. Knowledge is power.

Review the full list of medicines that you currently put in your body. As you get healthier, your need for potentially harmful substances will decrease, and so you should review that list with your physician. As your body regenerates and renews itself, you may find yourself able to eliminate medications that were previously necessary.

Ask for a full lipid profile to assess your cardio-metabolic risk (risk for heart disease) and also your hs-CRP to see your current state of inflammation. (This test will tell if your body is releasing substances that can damage your vessels and joints and age you prematurely.) Most importantly, keep this book with you as your health guide and refer to it on your journey to a healthier you. Some books change your life; this one could save it. Be mindful of every step. If you do just a few of the steps contained here, your health should increase exponentially.

Have appropriate cancer screenings. See the chart below:

YOUR CANCER SCREENING GUIDE FOR LIFELONG HEALTH

- **Breast:** self-exam monthly, doctor exam once or twice a year, first mammogram at age 35-40, then annually after 40.
- **Cervical:** first Pap smear at age 21 or within three years of sexual activity.
- **Colon:** first colonoscopy at age 50, then every ten years. Hemoccult test every five years.
- **Prostate:** digital exam and PSA yearly after age 39.
- **Skin:** self-exam regularly for unusual growing moles or lesions. Dermatologist once or twice annually for skin review. They have some cool new photographic mapping that can follow your skin health over time.

Get a baseline TSH to assess your thyroid function if you are female and over thirty-five. I recommend (although not everyone agrees) that you get up-to-date on your immunizations, including (ask your physician): pneumovax, tetanus, whooping cough, and influenza.

Ask your physician if you should start taking 75 milligrams of aspirin daily. The literature continues to report more and more benefits of its anti-inflammatory properties. Aspirin may have the ability to decrease the risk for stroke, but in those at risk, there is a growing body of information that low-dose aspirin reduces the risk of dying of a variety of cancers—gastrointestinal cancers, prostate cancer, lung cancer, with dramatic decrease in esophageal (60 percent) and colorectal (40 percent) cancers.

Note: The small but real risk of bleeding, especially internally, makes it paramount that you discuss aspirin with your physician before taking it.

GO TO YOUR DENTIST

Dental health is critical to obtain and maintain optimal health and is directly tied to your longevity. Maintaining your teeth and excellent gum health minimize inflammation and is part of the mind-set to optimal health.

MAKE THESE CHOICES:

- Brush at least twice a day with fluoride toothpaste.
- Floss daily.
- Have a yearly dental checkup.
- Have your teeth cleaned twice a year.
- Avoid all tobacco products.
- Minimize alcohol intake.
- Use lip balm that contains sunscreen.
- Combat dry mouth and keep your mouth and throat moist by chewing sugar-free gum, drinking water, and staying well hydrated.

. . .

These simple guidelines are foundational tools to keep you out of harm's way, protect you from potential invaders, and give you a checklist of preventative measures that can help you live a longer, healthier life. There are some actions that you are now going to take that you may have not done in the past. Everyone needs to be reminded once in awhile.

The benefits of my recommendations above are well documented in the medical literature. These very simple measures save hundreds of thousands of lives a year in the United States alone. Why fight the statistics? Lay the foundation for a healthy life, which will lead to longevity. Then layer the habits of health on top of that foundation to increase your vitality, energy, and lifestyle, and to decrease chances for disease.

In the next chapter, I am going to focus on the habits of health and the journey to create the skills, strategies, and tools to make optimal health a reality.

CHAPTER 10

Creating Your Healthy New World

> The awareness that health is dependent
> upon habits that we control makes us
> the first generation in history that to a
> large extent determines its own destiny.[1]
>
> —Jimmy Carter

I N THIS CHAPTER, WE WILL EXPLORE the important skills for adopting long-lasting change. As President Carter remarked, we know how important changing our behavior is to our country's health. Now you know how important it is to changing the trajectory of your own health.

Emerson once said, "The law of nature is do the thing, and you shall have the power." In order to find the tremendous treasure of long-term health that eludes most, you have to go from understanding to living the habits of health. The educator Horace Mann said, "Habit is a cable; we weave a thread of it each day, and at last we cannot break it." Our goal is not to break the long-term behaviors that have spun habits like thick cables. There is not enough willpower to overcome the continual forces of your previous programming and the obesegenic world you are exposed to daily. So instead you are going to develop a whole array of new habits that will form the foundational steps for your optimal health.

The first is to change your underlying environment to create a microenvironment of health.

1. CONSTRUCT YOUR HEALTHY NEW WORLD

Do you live in a food desert? That's a district in an urban or rural setting with few large grocery stores that offer the fresh and affordable foods needed to maintain a healthy diet. If you live in such an area, the impact on your health is substantial. If you have a normal grocery store but buy only processed food, you are creating a food desert in your own home.

> You've got bad eating habits if you use a grocery cart in 7-Eleven.[2]
>
> —Dennis Miller

The logistics of our lives sometimes forces us to take a shortcut. The quickest way to grab something to eat is to respond to what's immediately accessible—what is right in front of us. Humans are just wired that way. We become even more reactionary when we are busy and put in more hours at work. We react, instead of acting mindfully. It's the same way with everything in life, not just food. If we have a TV in our bedrooms, we will turn it on because it's there. If there's chocolate cake in the house, chances are someone's going to eat it.

So the first thing is to surround yourself with the best possible conditions for success.

Your Health Begins at Home

There is no place like home. It is a safe place where we spend more time than any other. If that's not a true statement for you and you work more hours than you spend at home, your life is upside down. But, with a little effort, you can quickly adjust to align your life and home environment with your goal for a healthier you. Here are some suggestions:

MODIFY YOUR SURROUNDINGS:

- Create a safe, healthy environment.
- Eliminate toxic foods, cleaning supplies, and other poisons such as radon.
- Ensure your water is clean.
- Ensure your air is clean.
- Check your smoke detectors to make sure they are working.
- Cover or fence your swimming pool.
- Eliminate potential hazards that could cause falls.
- Lock all doors when you are home.
- Lock up or eliminate firearms.
- Eliminate chemicals from your landscaping.

CREATE A KITCHEN MAKEOVER

- One of your first steps in learning to eat healthy for life is to learn proper portion size.
- Put away your large plates and bowls and replace them with nine-inch plates and cup-size bowls. Use only small forks and spoons.
- Use a food scale and measuring cups to regulate portion size.
- Place the proper amount of food onto your plate in the kitchen and then leave the kitchen and sit in the dining room. Don't place serving dishes on the table that may tempt you to take a second helping.
- Turn off the TV, which will decrease passive grazing and offer the opportunity for some real conversation with the family.
- Consider painting your kitchen blue and using blue plates and place mats. The color blue is known to decrease appetite while yellow and red increase it. (Why do you think McDonald's golden arches are the color they are?) uh-oh!
- Keep the lights on. Studies show that we tend to eat less in bright light.

KITCHEN CHECKLIST

✓ Food scale

✓ Measuring cups

✓ Small cups and bowls

⬜ 7- to 9-inch dinner plates

⬜ Teaspoons and salad forks *No*

⬜ Blue place mats and plates

✓ Bright lights

⬜ Refrigerator and cupboard makeover

Make it easy to avoid high-calorie, high-fat meals and snacks by getting rid of the following:

⬜ Whole-fat dairy products (whole milk, cheese, yogurt, cottage cheese, butter, and mayonnaise)

⬜ Processed deli meats

⬜ Fattening salad dressings

⬜ White bread, pasta, rice, and flour

⬜ Fruit drinks

⬜ Cookies, pastries, desserts

Don't use this exercise as a last chance to eat all the Oreo cookies left in the bag. Instead, give away foods to a neighbor or food bank. Once you get to your healthy weight, you can have an occasional Oreo if you want it. (Ninety-five percent of our taste satisfaction comes in the first three bites.)

REFRIGERATOR AND CUPBOARD CHECKLIST

Now restock your fridge and cupboards with these:

- Fat-free or low-fat dairy products (skim milk, low-fat yogurt, low-fat cheese)
- Lean proteins (skinless chicken, turkey breast, fish)
- Whole-grain bread and pasta, brown rice
- Beans
- Fresh fruits and vegetables
- Olive oil, vinegar, spray-type salad dressings
- Herbs and spices
- If necessary, choose one cupboard for other family members to use for their foods that aren't on your list. Better yet, ask them to join you in putting an end to unhealthy eating habits.

HEALTHY SNACKS

Replace high-calorie foods like peanuts and chips with fruits and fresh green vegetables. Here are some great low-calorie snacks:

- Asparagus (1/2 cup = 18 calories, 3 carbohydrates)
- Broccoli (1 cup = 44 calories, 8 carbohydrates)
- Sugar-free Jell-O (1 Snack Cup = 10 calories, 0 carbohydrates)
- Cauliflower (2 oz. = 12 calories, 2 carbohydrates)
- Celery (1 stalk = 6 calories, 1 carbohydrates)
- Dill pickle (1 = 4 calories, 1 carbohydrates)
- Radishes (1 oz. = 8 calories, 2 carbohydrates)
- Spinach (1 cup = 6 calories, 1 carbohydrates)
- Bouillon (1 cup = 10 calories, 1 carbohydrates)
- Cucumber (1 cup = 15 calories, 3 carbohydrates)
- Lettuce (1 cup = 2 calories, 0 carbohydrates)

Before you grab something to eat, make sure you are actually hungry and not just thirsty. Approximately 30 percent of the time, thirst is disguised as hunger. Try drinking a big glass of water and wait ten minutes. Then rate your hunger on a scale of one to ten; you may not need that snack after all. This example shows how being mindful can help you develop the habits of health.

Your Bedroom Makeover

Studies show that sleep is key to not just your overall health, but your ability to lose and maintain a healthy weight. That is why it is so important to get at least seven hours of sleep a night.

Design your bedroom for relaxation by using calming colors. If brown seems more restful to you, use beige and brown tones. If peach, yellow, or lavender makes you feel calm, use those colors. Revamp your bedroom for comfort. Use relaxing scents, if that helps. Stay away from late night TV and read a motivational book instead, or write your day's activity in your journal. Get rid of the clutter in your bedroom and in your closets by taking all those clothes that are too big for you to the consignment shop.

BEDROOM HEALTHY CHECKLIST

- Remove your TV.
- Decorate with soft calming colors.
- Bring your journal to bed for your evening entry to review what you did right and what you could have done better.
- Keep your bedroom neat.
- Use scented candles or potpourri.
- Play calming music.
- Keep motivating books on your nightstand or on your iPad.
- Learn how to shut down the phones and tablets for nighttime.
- Get at least seven to eight hours sleep.

Your Work Environment

If you work for yourself or from your home (which I highly recommend), then you completely control your work environment. If you work in an office, you have more of a challenge, but there are many small modifications that can improve that office space as well. Do anything you can to create a relaxing work space with colors, decorations, flowers, soft music, and personal pictures to build a peaceful environment. Immediately remove all candies and unhealthy snack foods. This eliminates any temptations you face after stress. The key is to make it easy to succeed, not to make it easy to fail.

If you are physically able to, replace your chair with a ball chair, which is literally a large rubber ball on a stable base. If you must sit, this will allow you to constantly work on your core and burn calories at the same time. Another great way to get you off your rear is by using a headset so you can talk on the phone while standing up. These helpful modifications reduce sitting time. If you're standing, you're likely to stretch often. If you're sitting on a ball, you're likely to sit up straight and align your spine with better posture.

WORK CHECKLIST

- Clear out all unhealthy food from desktop and drawers.
- Consider getting a ball chair.
- Use a headset for your phone so you can stand while talking.
- Change restroom and water cooler usage to the farthest practical location.
- Soften the work environment with personal touches.

Your Relationship Makeover

Whatever herd you hang out with is the herd you'll become most like. If you're a cow, you graze. If you're a duck, you swim. If you're a sea-gull, you fly. Whatever group you choose will usually determine your behavior, simply because you're with them frequently. Choose wisely. Albert Bandura of Stanford University did some powerful research on behavior modification.[3] He revolutionized our understanding of how observation of others influences our behavior. It is one of the most important factors in changing health behaviors and critical in maintain-ing the changes.

For example, hanging out with people living my habits of health helps me stay focused and make the right choices. At the beginning of the decade, I created a health network focused on health as a priority. It has been a critical part of both implementing and supporting long-term success. Not only has this healthy community aided me in helping thousands of people create long-term optimal health, but it has also been essential for me personally.

The *New England Journal of Medicine* in July 2007 published a social study that confirmed the spread of obesity through associations, even if the relationships were not in the same geographical surroundings.[4] So my first question for you is, how healthy are your five closest friends? If the answer is not very healthy, you may have to put those relationships on hold for a while. I am not talking about a divorce, but start looking for people who have the same desire as you for making health a priority. Name five people you know who are actively working toward optimal health in their own lives and think of some ways you can spend more time with them.

My second question is, how healthy is your surrounding com-munity? If you are spending your time at happy hour or football tailgates, you may want to consider a different path. Are there community recrea-tion centers, gyms, parks, or fitness groups you can join?

HEALTHY RELATIONSHIP CHECKLIST

- Go for a walk in your community, and if you have a dog, take him with you (a healthier dog will be your first healthy friend).
- Meet other health-minded walkers.
- Join a community recreation center.
- Join a gym.
- Sign up for a sporting event either as a participant, if you are ready, or as an observer, if you are not ready.
- Join an activity group, for example, a Pilates group.

2. ESTABLISH A STRONG SUPPORT NETWORK

In the first section, I suggested necessary adjustments to your home and surrounding environment. Here I want to address some of the ways you can develop your own support system for reducing stress (in all quadrants of your life) and managing your health, starting with your immediate family and friends. You will of course work directly with your physician to manage any current health challenges.

One of your biggest mistakes is to start out on this journey by yourself. You simply don't have all the answers, and even if you did, you need a strong emotional network of friends, family, and health-minded professionals in your corner. You simply can't do it yourself.

Approximately 80 percent of disease is linked to some kind of stress. Physical stress taxes the organs, inhibits blood flow, causes spikes in blood pressure, and increases chances for heart disease, stroke, and diabetes. Physical stress caused by excess weight or an unhealthy diet compounds year after year until your body becomes a ticking time bomb. Emotional stressors (if left unmanaged) exacerbate the problem. Managing physical and emotional stress and understanding the triggers are critical. Our obesegenic chaotic world is a formable opponent in the fight for your health. Pile on top of that the stress of relationships, deadlines, seemingly endless work schedules, and to-do lists, and there is good reason that most people fail in changing their health habits and their health.

Getting healthy can be contagious, so ask your family and friends if they want to start on the journey with you. If they are not interested, ask them to please support you, because it's important to you.

If you join forces on this journey to optimal health with your spouse, significant other, or a close friend, you are more likely to be successful. Having a partner or friend who also is intrinsically motivated to create health can really fuel and maintain your success.

In an Australian study, researchers found that couples who changed their behavior as a team were more successful than people going it alone. The couples' lifestyle was not only healthier, but they were more likely at one year to maintain the healthy lifestyle.[5]

Also a British study of almost 1500 couples participating in a lifestyle intervention program to reduce the risk of heart disease found that those who benefited the most had partners who also benefited the most.[6]

So having your spouse join you can certainly be helpful, and if you are successful they are more likely to be successful. Of course, it only works if he or she makes the decision because he or she wants to. You can certainly help awaken that desire by creating a rationale that explains why making the change is important. (Have them read this book.) Also it may be helpful in overcoming your partner's resistance to acknowledge that they may not want to do it and then inviting them to join you so you can do it together.

But if they don't, go for it anyway and get healthy!

Once you really have decided to create health, and you tell those around you, it has a power in itself. The momentum builds, and other health-minded people will be drawn to you. You'll discover others just by virtue of your new physical activity, and you'll find there are resources if you want to join clubs, groups, or even online coaching or fitness and nutrition programs that support your health goals.

Many people find that a professional coach who is solely vested in their success can be helpful if they are having difficulty getting going or staying on track with new healthy habits. Whatever works for you and your life is the best way to go. Just be mindful of your triggers, habits, strengths, weaknesses, and needs.

The best approach is to combine aspects of the different support systems that work for your own life, scheduling, time, and personality. A study from the *Annals of Internal Medicine* compared three approaches to lifestyle intervention for producing weight loss in diabetic patients.[7] The three approaches were a coach-led intervention, a patient self-directed DVD intervention, and what the study referred to as "usual care."

The coach-led intervention produced the best results, followed by the self-directed DVD group, both of which outperformed "usual care," which meant having a patient try to lose weight on his own. Why did the coach-led intervention achieve the best results? A patient having a coach is no different than a world-class Olympic athlete or a professional golfer having a coach. If athletes who compete at the highest levels need one, patients can certainly benefit, too. Accountability helps you achieve your goals.

HEALTHY SUPPORT SYSTEM CHECKLIST

- Think of 5 people you know who are focused on health.
- Let them know that you are choosing health as well.
- Find ways to connect and start activities.
- Check out health support groups in churches, community centers, or online.
- Work with a health coach. If you already have one, tell him or her you are asking for help. If you are looking for one, go to my website and fill out the questionnaire. We will connect you with a coach.
- Ask your doctor.

There are lists of resources you can refer to in the appendix. You can also go to my website at www.habitsofhealth.net for online support and resources.

3. PUT YOURSELF AT THE CENTER

I have discussed preparing your environment and establishing a support structure for the best possible chance for success. Since you have decided to create health, there is no pressure from the outside. Now it's time to place yourself in the middle of this new healthy structure. Put up your optimal health story board in a prominent place in your home. Get up each day making mindful decisions.

It's all about your choices. You can wake up every morning and decide whether to eat a healthy breakfast or no breakfast at all. If you are on a meal replacement plan such as the one we offer at Take Shape For Life, you can either follow it religiously or not; it's your choice. You can decide to use either the stairs or the elevator when you get to work. The choice is yours. You are the dominant force in your life.

Minimizing negative habits will help increase your longevity and healthy habits. However, if you do make a negative choice, don't beat yourself up. Instead, evaluate why it occurred. Were you tired, stressed, or just feeling lazy? Understanding what drives decisions is an important part of the process. What could you have done differently? Improving each and every day is part of the process, until it becomes easy to make healthy choices.

Record your progress in your journal once you're on the path to creating new healthy habits. Write about what worked and what didn't. Journaling is a powerfully useful tool because it gives you a great reference point for your progress. When you write down where you've been, you can see how far you've gone and how much you've achieved. Journaling helps you express and unload emotions—by writing them down—instead of responding to emotions in unhealthy ways.

Journaling is an internal process, but combined with peers, coaches, counselors, and people with similar goals and orientation, you create a powerful community of influence to help increase your habits of health.

You can text, tweet, e-mail, call, share pictures on Pinterest, and engage in the habits of health by association and continuous action. You can talk about it when you are at the gym, at work, on a walk with neighbors, or while doing a 5K walk for charity.

Your focus on reaching your optimal health will start driving your decisions. You are intrinsically motivated to do it. As you get better and better, you will want to tell others and share the benefits you have realized. The habits of health will expand your mind and your life.

I've added a thirty-day challenge that will connect you to the habits of health with daily e-mails that you can sign up for by going to www.habitsofhealth.net. The more ways you can become connected and focused on health the better.

YOU ARE LIVING THE HABITS OF HEALTH

- Display your optimal health board and declare that you are open for business—the business of becoming as healthy as possible.
- Choose to conduct every day as you decide to.
- Be mindfully healthy.
- Work on increasing the pluses and decreasing the minuses.
- Plug into your support system wih texting, tweeting, e-mails, Pinterest, phone calls, and groups.
- Reach out to others, because it's important to stay connected and get better and stronger.

As you put yourself on the path toward this goal, you may experience doubts along the way, so let's discuss the mind, which is the key programmer of everything we do.

4. PRACTICE MINDFULNESS
AND RELAXATION

Obsessing about the past and worrying about the future keeps us from paying attention to the most important time, the present. Stay focused on being mindful of this one moment. Find the space and time for quiet, peace, or solitude.

MOMENTS FOR YOURSELF

- Quiet time on a train
- Sitting in your garden
- Swimming in your pool
- Going for a walk along a body of water or in the woods
- Yoga
- Martial arts
- Meditation/prayer
- Time alone on a treadmill
- Escape to a park for lunch once a week
- Take up walking or running on a trail, instead of the road

Consider these questions:

- What techniques do you use now to create mindfulness?

- How many times a day do you create a moment of mindfulness?

- Are you aware of everything you put in your mouth, either food or liquid?

- Do you stop to taste every bite?

- Are you aware of your body's every move?

Cultivating natural awareness is very helpful in monitoring choices and making the necessary corrections to increase our positives. It also allows us to notice when something about our bodies has changed, so we can be the most advanced early warning system for potential problems.

In the quest to help you create optimal health, it's important to appreciate the mind-body connection. I'm not referring to a deep, metaphysical, spiritual journey, although that is certainly worth exploring as you head toward self-discovery.

Here I am talking about the simple fact that everything you see and hear and taste and feel and smell and think about has a direct effect on your body. The mind is connected to the body. What you put in the mind affects the stress levels and chemistry of the body. What you put in the body can affect the mind. Good, healthy food helps you think better, digest better, and concentrate better. Heavy, processed foods can clog your arteries and slow down circulation and concentration.

By becoming aware when you are drifting off into unhealthy decisions, you can improve your self-management. When you respond with conscious choice rather than automatically reacting the way you did in the past, you take the game to the next level. Here are some examples of conscious choices:

- Ninety-five percent of taste satisfaction comes in the first three bites. By tasting at that level, you can experience all the tastes you crave without the quantities that can harm you.

- At a cocktail party, instead of drinking three cocktails, you could order club soda with lime, which also keeps you from eating seventeen scallops wrapped in bacon.

- After a stressful meeting, you drive straight home and drink the specialty waters you have in your fridge instead of stopping for happy hour.

Consider these questions:

- What situations in the past have led you to overeat, drink too much, or smoke?

- Has this behavior been a recurring event?

- What could you have done differently if you increased your awareness?

One of the most important keys to creating long-term health is raising your level of self-awareness and mindfulness. Remember that your body is designed to store and conserve energy. But if you go through your day on automatic, your programming will add a lot of negatives in the form of energy-dense calories.

The default program for early humans was the parasympathetic nervous system. Their normal state was calm, with a slow heart rate, high degree of alertness, and body organs functioning very efficiently. When a real threat presented itself, such as a saber-toothed tiger, the emotional area would switch to a high sympathetic outflow of cortisol, epinephrine, and norepinephrine, and humans would run like the wind.

The body ate up all these chemicals as they fueled the muscles, heart, and circulation. Today, we are stressed and in a high sympathetic state with all those chemicals circulating (and not being used), because the threats are not real and there is nothing to run from. We sit at our desks or in a meeting, while those chemicals increase inflammation, raise insulin, prematurely age us, and cause blood pressure to rise. Reaching a high state of health is impossible unless you can control your mind. Lower your stress level by doing relaxation exercises.

Stress Reduction

When I coach people through the process of reducing stress, I give them a technique called the relaxation response. This technique was developed by Dr. Herbert Benson at Harvard and involves teaching the neocortex to relax.[8] How does it work? It turns off the cycle of continual thoughts that invade your mind and your subconscious, and impede your progress.

These automatic thoughts are not productive. Here's how to do the relaxation response:

1. Set aside ten to twenty minutes.

2. Find a quiet place where you can be alone.

3. Sit up straight, in a comfortable relaxed position.

4. Close your eyes and release any tension. Stay in the moment.

5. Turn off your brain. Eliminate all thoughts and create a blank slate. Think about one word, such as love, peace, or power, and meditate on it.

6. Keep repeating that word, then sit quietly for a minute or two, exhale, breathe, and relax.

You've just achieved a new state of composure and control. Here are some other ways you can control your stress:

STRATEGIES TO LOWER YOUR INTERNAL STRESS

DEEP BREATHING: breathe in deep through your nose. Stop. Be mindful and aware. Exhale. Breathing deep is one of the fastest ways to relieve stress.

PRAYER: go to a quiet place like the park, a patch of grass under a tree, or even just the bathroom. It doesn't have to be the idyllic location. God is everywhere. Take a moment to stop, release yourself, talk to God, and realize you may not have all the answers.
If you are agnostic, then talk to whoever gives you guidance.

YOGA/STRETCHING: the body reaps amazing benefits when your muscles are stretched. Relax over a large workout ball. Bend backwards and stretch out your spine. If you don't have one, buy one! Attend a yoga class, use a DVD at home, or stretch on the floor every night. Stretching elongates muscles and releases the tension.

A recent study shows that mindfulness meditation dramatically lowers the inflammatory markers of stress and is an important exercise to protect our bodies.[9]

5. TAME YOUR INNER SELF

Each of us is the culmination of our experiences, mentorship, and environment. First realize that you are unique among humans. Your past has influenced not just your physical health but also your mental health. How you respond to both your inner world and your outer world is unique.

Your life started simply in your interaction with the environment. Your response when you needed something or didn't like something was the same. You cried and somebody took care of you. You were completely dependent. Through your development, you became socialized by people who, I hope, loved and cared for you. During this time, you learned to manage your world.

But the crying technique that works so well for infants will not work for adult interactions in daily life. So, in this section, I am going to discuss emotional intelligence. Your emotional intelligence is your ability to recognize and understand your emotions and manage your responses and interactions with others.

Less than 40 percent of the population can identify their emotions as they occur. In order to manage our emotions, we must first identify them. People who improve their emotional intelligence have better control over their lives, habits, and unhealthy behaviors.

Let's start with you and your emotions.

Are You Aware of Your Emotions?

Emotions, as I mentioned earlier, can be broken down into five key categories. Happiness, sadness, anger, fear, and shame are the basic feelings from which many variations are derived. As we go though our day, we constantly experience a full range of feelings. We are always reacting to something, not just in a cognitive way, but also in an emotional way. This is where mindfulness can immediately start serving you. Make sure you are mindful and pay full attention during your next interaction with someone. What emotions are you feeling? Start taking an interest in your inner world. When you feel uneasiness, have an increasing heart rate, are flushed, or have a funny feeling in your stomach, I want you to:

STOP

- Refocus on the exact moment.

- Now ask yourself what you are feeling.

- Do not try to analyze it; just become aware.

- Do that for the next couple of days.

This exercise is the most important new skill to refine. You will soon realize that your first reaction to almost everything around you is an emotional one. That is how your brain processes every move in your interactions in the world.

> The flight response was critical to humans' survival 10,000 years ago. Less thinking meant more action. Watch a bird at a feeder. It may be eating, but it is constantly looking up and around. If anything startles it, it takes immediate flight.
>
> Notice when you get upset. You may feel anger and show poor thinking that clouds your judgment. When you have an intense emotional response, you cannot think clearly.
>
> When a child becomes upset while learning to read, she is no longer able to focus.
>
> **People go from learning to reacting.**

Pay attention to how you are processing and how your emotions *affect* your thought process.

Are You Regulating Your Response to Your Emotions?

Notice how you have no control over your feelings. *You feel what you feel. You do have control over the thoughts that follow and complete control of how you react to those emotions.* This reflective period when you decide to interpret what the emotion means and how you respond gives you power and control over your health and your life.

Now I want you to add another step after Stop in the previous exercise:

CHALLENGE

Evaluate why you are feeling a certain way. Are you afraid because there is a scary man walking behind you, or are you scared because you just stepped on a crack in the sidewalk? The former serves you well by increasing your level of awareness and avoidance; the latter is a neurosis and superstition not based on reality. It causes harmful anxiety and, if it leads to eating a candy bar, it creates minuses in your health trajectory.

After evaluating why you are feeling what you are feeling and determining real versus imagined threats, add another step:

CHOOSE

Here is the most important part of changing your health world. By choosing the response that best serves you in the long run, you will become better at avoiding those bad choices. Triggers, which are prolonged emotional feelings, can no longer stimulate you to eat the candy bar or smoke the cigarette. You no longer are a pawn to your emotions. Someone who challenges your intelligence or your self-worth no longer causes a reactive outburst followed by unhealthy behaviors.

> **An easy way to stop letting people push our buttons is to ask:**
>
> What am I not getting in this situation? That is, respect or recognition.
>
> Do I really need it?
>
> Do I really need this person to think I am smart, or pretty?
>
> If I really do need it, then there is a more appropriate way to resolve it than having a temper tantrum.
>
> **And if it's just my ego, let it go!**

Now you have a powerful tool to help you become aware, challenge, and regulate your emotions. With mindfulness and practice, you will be able to control your habits of disease, and as a result of decreasing your stress, you will improve your health directly.

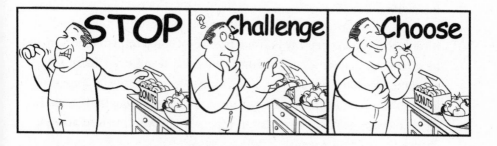

Understanding how those around you are feeling and how you can improve your relationships is also important.

Are You Aware of Your Interactions with Others?

Your ability to better understand what others are feeling and why they are responding in a certain way is very important in enhancing your health and well-being. It goes back to mindfulness and staying focused on what is going on around you. By listening, observing, and becoming better at looking at a situation through *someone else's* vantage point, you will influence how you will better manage your time together.

The next time you enter a social situation, observe others' body language and the mood of the room. Look for things in the room you have never noticed. By being observant and sensing the dynamics present, you will be able to communicate more effectively, with less chance of creating an unwanted emotion, drama, or unhealthy situation or crisis.

How Do You Handle Your Relationships?

Your ability to develop and maintain strong relationships is based on consistency in communications and in behavior. Great friendships and relationships are not only highly desirable to manage our interactions effectively but are also associated with well-being.

In my book, *Dr. A's Habits of Health*, I interviewed and did extensive research on people who live to be over a hundred years of age in great health. Among the most important factors are their deep, long-term relationships. You should seek and covet these associations and develop those precious relationships. That requires work and results from spending meaningful time, especially in times of stress. Casual acquaintances may be supportive under normal conditions but collapse in a stressful situation. Since modern life is full of stress, it is critical to manage stressful occasions. Your ability to be aware of and regulate your own emotions and correctly sense and understand your relationships will give you the best possible chance to correctly negotiate a difficult situation.

The next time you sense that a conversation is going to become confrontational, follow these steps:

STOP—CHALLENGE—CHOOSE

- What am I feeling? Why?

- Am I acknowledging the other person's feelings?

- Am I being open?

- Am I giving advice or actually working to resolve amicably?

- Or am I letting my ego take over?

- Am I showing how much I care?

Developing your emotional control and managing yourself and your relationships takes time. But the payoff is very important as you seek to create optimal health. Your mind controls your body. You want your mind and your relationships to be "at ease," not progressing down the path to "dis-ease."

You now have the five core pieces necessary to make the habits of health a part of you.

In the next chapter, I will discuss how to fully integrate optimal health into your life. These elements will help solidify the habits of health as a part of your internal life every day. Just as the working parts of an engine make up the whole, these components of intrinsic desire and external action combine to help create a healthier mind and body.

CHAPTER 11

Integrating the Habits of Health into Your Life

Things start out as hopes and end up as habits.[1]

—Lillian Hellman

Optimal health is a journey taken one step, one habit, and one day at a time.

—Dr. Wayne Scott Andersen

CONGRATULATIONS! YOU ARE WELL SUPPLIED with the building blocks for progressive success. If someone can overcome psychological and logistical barriers, he or she can overcome obesity and poor health in only months. We have spent ten chapters focusing on that goal. Together we have created a healthy environment in you and around you. You now have a thorough understanding of the process necessary to create optimal health in your life.

We now begin your integration by introducing some of the key building blocks of optimal health. This is the starting point of a complete process for the rest of your life. You will take the habits of health and internalize them into every fabric of your being so that they become your standard operating procedure.

The path to optimal health will be a bit inconvenient for a while, filled with simple, mundane, insignificant choices, and will challenge you. You are taking responsibility, getting out of your comfort zone; you are swimming against many who appear to be deceptively comfortable. They may be comfortable on their couches or at the fast-food restaurants now, but they will become less comfortable later. Inconvenience will creep in and eventually dominate their every moment. They will endure daily life with low energy, chronic pain, and lack of libido, medication's side effects, and many trips to the bathroom nightly. The highlight of the week will be multiple doctor appointments and the haunting reality that each morning they must struggle through another day.

Mindfully, you are making very different choices, which are the small, daily disciplines that lead to health. Watch those around you eating those fries and drinking those sodas, unaware that their bodies are on slow discharge, the way your cell phone no longer functions if you leave it on.

Your path will be very different.

THE PATH AND THE TOOLS

As you start on the path to full integration, you won't notice a huge difference immediately, but understand that the positive effects are being set in motion. The implementation of the habits of health strategy, blueprint, and tools assure you are on the right path. I have provided you with the operating instructions to reach optimal health. If you just have patience, you will notice the differences.

The secret ingredient is *time*. The immediate effect of most of those small adjustments is almost undetectable, yet some of the habits of health will have an almost immediate noticeable effect.

Among the areas of rapid improvement, two are worth a moment of discussion here. They are both key habits of health.

First as we focus on the habits of healthy weight loss, I will discuss the use of meal replacements as a tool that can create very efficient, safe weight loss. Because they make a difference almost immediately, I find them very powerful in creating a generative, teachable moment. The progressive weight reduction reinforces health and vitality when the burden of being overweight is removed. Over time, when combined with other healthy eating choices, they can help you develop the habits of healthy eating for life.

These tools are catalysts that, by design, help your body in its recovery. They work with your body to empty your overstuffed fat cells in a safe, effective fashion. The cells empty, eliminating unhealthy substances that affect your blood pressure and blood sugar and that have myriad other harmful effects.

Another rapid improvement may be made in the area of healthy sleep. You may notice improvement in your sleep soon after you remove the TV from your bedroom. Remove the stimulation, and the mind is free to drift rapidly into latency. The result is deep, restoring REM cycles that occur naturally, rather than insomnia from an overactive mind preoccupied with defeating the space invader viewed at bedtime.

Yes, a few of these health-changing habits bring immediate benefits. But the majority of your new choices will show their health-generating effects in a more subtle fashion.

The hundreds of other small disciplines that you also progressively add to your daily choices in all areas of your health, when repeated every day, make the *most* difference. You will have to be focused to build these new habits of health, because these small things are easy to do or not do. Since the health benefits won't show up until later, you have to be disciplined to do them because you do not get that immediate feedback of improvement. Some effects will reveal themselves in weeks; some not until years later. A recent study by the Cooper Institute showed a dramatic reduction in dementia later in life for those who were fit in their fifties.[2] The benefits from their healthy choices didn't show up until twenty years later.

The graph at the beginning of chapter 8 illustrating the trajectory of your daily choices shows the effect of all the little positives that separate you from your past state of health over time. You are now harnessing time as your friend. There is no steady state in the trajectory of life. Either you are getting healthier or you are getting sicker. Most people focus on the past, which actually pulls them toward disease. That focus makes no sense, because you can only change the future.

There is only one way you can fill your future with radiant health. It is to focus on your choices in the moment, through your newfound skills of mindfulness and knowing the right choices. You have made a fundamental choice to get healthier. You have set your gyroscope pointing directly toward your optimal health. Now I will help you begin filling in all those changes in choice. I am going to take the necessary parts for optimal health and assemble them into a comprehensive strategy specifically to meet your logistical and psychological needs for long-term success.

CREATE YOUR MASTER PLAN
USING STRUCTURAL DYNAMICS

First construct a structure to advance you toward your goals. The structure is kind of like a GPS system. It will give you an awareness of your current position on the health continuum and direct you toward your desired destination, optimal health. The construction begins when you answer two questions: Where are you now? Where do you want to go?

Where Are You Now?

In chapter 2, you filled out a questionnaire. Your answers placed you at a point on the health continuum. Here are some of those key areas that helped you identify your current health status:

DESCRIBE YOUR CURRENT HEALTH STATUS

Smoke:	Yes		No	
Weight:	Obese	Overweight	Normal	
Eat Healthy:	No	Sometimes	Always	Not Sure
Activity Level:	None	Low	Medium	Heavy
Sleep Hours:	Very Low <5	Low 5 to 6	Normal 7 to 8	High >8
Sleep Quality:	Poor	Fair	Good	Excellent
Stress Level:	Extreme	High	Medium	Low	None

What is your position on this chart?

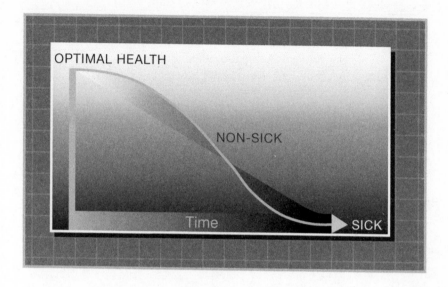

Where Do You Want to Go?

In chapter 7, you wrote down your desired health outcomes. You created a visual representation with your optimal health story board, which is an important tool to help you integrate. A recent study reinforces the power of using visual images, such as an optimal health story board, in improving the health of very overweight children.[3]

To get you started, I have listed many of the basic, desired health outcomes. Now, let's put together your desired outcome and your current reality to create a structural tension chart or master plan for creating health.

DESIRED OUTCOME:

Optimal Health

Non-Smoker, Normal Weight, Eat Healthy,
Activity Level High, High Quality Sleep of 7–8 hours,
Stress Level: Low or none

SECONDARY CHOICE   TIME COMPLETE

Habits of Healthy Eating

Habits of Motion

Habits of Healthy Sleep

Habits of a Healthy Mind

Habits of Well-being

Current Reality

CIRCLE YOUR CURRENT HEALTH STATUS
Smoke: Yes or No
Weight: Obese, Overweight, Normal
Eat Healthy: No, Sometimes, Always, Not Sure
Activity Level: None, Low, Medium, Heavy
Sleep Hours: Very Low <5, Low 5 to 6, Normal 7 to 8, High >8
Sleep Quality: Poor, Fair, Good, Excellent
Stress Level: Extreme, High, Medium, Low, None

As well as you can, fill in the specific health challenges you have now, including medications, disease, and unhealthy lab results, if known. The more specific you can be about your current reality, the better. The same goes for your desired outcomes. Make sure you are not writing down processes, but actual outcomes. For example, "I will run three days a week" is a process. Ask yourself what running three days a week will accomplish. Instead, as an outcome, you could say "cardio-vascular fitness."

Be bold with your desired outcomes. They are not what you think you can do but what you really want. They should be realistic but represent the best you can be.

As you can see, the choices on the left side of the master plan are big foundational pieces of your health that will take some time to become completely integrated. You will look back in the future with great satisfaction as you have mastered each one of them and others that you will add as you progress on your optimal health journey.

We will now focus on how to break them down into manageable bite-size pieces that can be added in baby steps to your day.

FIVE KEY HABITS OF HEALTH (SECONDARY CHOICES)

The secondary choices are the action steps that will move you toward your optimal health goals. In the master structural tension chart, I chose five key habits of health that are essential for reaching and maintaining optimal health. We will start your integration in those key areas throughout the rest of the book. With your new optimal health master plan, you will now be able to break down all of the secondary choices or action steps in the various foundational pieces of your health. These choices will expand as you gain competence and master your health as you become fully integrated. (As I mentioned, my close friend, colleague, and mentor Robert Fritz has pioneered this work on the creative process.)

I find having a master plan extremely important in helping generate the momentum to move you toward your goals. By placing yourself in the center of this dynamic, you can always focus on where you want to go and the steps to get you there. Also, by having due dates, you create an urgency that will help you find the secondary action steps to achieve your goal.

I outline here the steps for creating a basic structural tension chart. You will use this in the following chapters to create your unique plan in the foundational areas we will be discussing in detail. It is the same process we used to develop your master optimal health plan. I hope you will use the process in organizing all of your health and life goals. Understanding structural dynamics is an important part of preventing oscillation and yo-yoing, which can derail your progress. Structural tension is an integral part of the habits of health system. You should master it in order to reach your fundamental choice of optimal health. (For a much more detailed study, please go to www.robertfritz.com, where you can find online courses, books, and other instruction on the creative process.)

Creating a Structural Tension Chart

Step 1: What is your desired outcome?
It should be a clear, visual, outcome that you desire, not a process to get you there:

        Desired outcome: _____

Step 2: What is the current reality in relationship to your desired outcome?

        Current reality: _____

Step 3: Write the desired outcome and the current reality on your chart and simultaneously visualize it in your mind.
Visualize your desired outcome at the same time you become aware of your current location on the chart. As you focus on the desired outcome for some aspect of your health (and life) and know where you currently are, it creates a generative momentum toward that goal.

Step 4: Write down action steps or secondary choices that support your primary vision or goal.

As you hold the tension between your desired outcome and your current realty in relation to that outcome, write down all the action steps that will move you toward that goal.

Step 5: Write down due dates that quantify when you will reach the different action steps or secondary choices that support your primary choice or desired outcome.

STRUCTURAL TENSION CHART

DESIRED OUTCOME: _____

ACTION STEPS
(SECONDARY CHOICE)

DUE DATES

_____   _____

_____   _____

_____   _____

_____   _____

_____

CURRENT REALITY: _____

You can use the structural tension charts to create all the different areas in your health and life. Making the new habits of health a lasting part of your life as you become an optimally healthy individual is a formula I call the "cycle of success."

The cycle starts by developing a clear understanding of the principle, secondary choice, or action step and then starting the action. You then review the results to make sure the actions are moving you toward your desired health outcomes. You then make the necessary corrections and repeat the action steps.

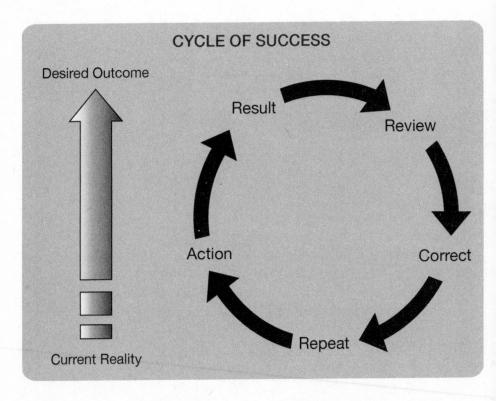

Now you have a powerful mechanism to help create the desired outcomes in the different foundational pieces. By developing a generative, dynamic structure that allows you to organize all the secondary choices and timelines, you can precisely focus on multiple building blocks of optimal health.

Becoming as healthy as possible is going to take some time. It is a journey that will continue for your whole, healthy life. We all start on this journey at different points in our lives, both chronologically and at different positions on the path to optimal health. Your master plan should start with some fundamental areas, which you will soon integrate into your optimal health plan and then ingrain the corresponding habits of health.

As you begin your integration process, you must first address two very common yet critical areas, which many of us struggle with, that will determine your success.

Two Fundamental Deal Breakers

There are two fundamental areas that you need to address immediately as part of your desire to create optimal health for yourself: smoking and your current weight (if your current weight and waist circumference place you at risk for disease).

SMOKING

When it comes to fundamental choices, if you don't quit cigarette smoking, your body has little chance of optimization. The direct and indirect negative impacts on your body leave no rational argument for continuing it, if you happen to still subscribe to this lethal habit of disease. I hope by now you understand that you have the power to resolve to become a nonsmoker. If you have a deep resolve to quit and are ready to fully endorse that decision, it should be your first area of focus. I highly suggest that you immediately schedule

An estimated 45.3 million people, or 19.3% of all adults (aged 18 years or older), in the United States smoke cigarettes.[4] Cigarette smoking is more common among men (21.5%) than women (17.3%).[4]

Cigarette smoking is the leading cause of preventable death in the United States,[5] accounting for approximately 443,000 deaths, or 1 of every 5 deaths, in the United States each year.[6,7]

Smoking affects almost 20% of the population and is the primary cause of preventable deaths in the U.S. Not far behind is obesity, which accounts for almost 300,000 deaths in the U.S. alone and affects over 30% of Americans and if you include those that are overweight is a staggering 67%.

an appointment with your physician. Tell him or her that you have made a fundamental decision to create health in your life and the first step is to stop smoking. In this book, I focus on helping you create what you want, not what you do not want. The specific techniques to stop smoking are beyond the scope of this book and may include medications, hypnosis, acupuncture, and specific counseling and focus groups, but the most important element of your success is you.

Use this book with its strategies, tools, skills, and techniques to help guide your success. Many people have told me that reading my books has had a major impact on helping them become nonsmokers.

YOUR CURRENT WEIGHT

To evaluate whether or not your weight is putting you at risk for disease, calculate your Body Mass Index and waist circumference. (Visit www.habitsofhealth.net for guidance or use the Body Mass Index chart in chapter 1.)

Are your BMI and waist circumference putting you at risk? If the answer is yes, in the next two chapters, I will help you integrate healthy weight loss to move you toward your goal to create optimal health. If you are already at a healthy weight, you can move on to chapter 13 and start integrating your healthy eating, which will help keep you at a healthy weight and help you focus on creating the best possible nutritional intake to reach optimal health.

BODY MASS INDEX

- < 25 Low risk
- 25 - 29.9 Moderate risk
- 30 - 35 High risk
- > 35 Extremely high risk

WAIST CIRCUMFERENCE:

- Male > 37 inches   Increase risk
- Female > 32 inches   Increase risk

. . .

Now you have a master plan and a powerful mechanism in structural tension to move your health on the trajectory of optimal health.

In the next five chapters, I introduce key areas of focus to help you fully integrate the habits necessary to lay a foundation for optimal health. These chapters are designed to help you *discover* your path to optimal health and begin your journey. They are intended to awaken your desire and start building your competencies so that you will want to progress to the comprehensive habits of health system.

CHAPTER 12

Discover the Habits of Healthy Weight Loss

A diet is a plan, generally hopeless, for reducing your weight, which tests your willpower but does little for your waistline.[1]

—**Herbert B. Prochnow**

A RE YOUR BMI AND WAIST CIRCUMFERENCE putting you at risk? The task of reaching a healthy weight is challenging because, unlike smoking or drinking alcohol, we have to eat. Yet if we stop looking at dieting as a thing we do to ourselves, but instead focus on creating a healthy weight to support the healthy person we become, it is a much easier undertaking. It is a key habit of health and worthy of your immediate attention and focus.

The literature is full of statistics and studies that support the importance of reaching a healthy weight and lifestyle in preventing disease and creating long-term health. (The notes section at the end of the book has further reading about how discovering and reaching optimal health can help you live a longer, healthier life.[2])

The great news is that by reducing your weight by 10 percent, you lower your risk for disease almost 50 percent. And the even better news, if you are overweight, is that I'm now your personal coach and I am very good at helping people lose weight (and even better at helping them keep it off through the habits of health).

YOUR ENERGY MANAGEMENT

Everyone comes into this world with specific genetic programming. You can thank your parents for whether that has helped or hurt you to this point. Genetics has probably had some effect on how well your body processes food and energy, as well as how much muscle mass you have. If you had overweight parents, you have a greater tendency to also be overweight. If you had skinny, tall parents, you are likely to be skinny and tall. However, that's not always the case, and it's not necessarily your destiny. The truth is that approximately 70 percent of your current weight is determined by how well you have managed your energy until now. It is a very simple relationship:

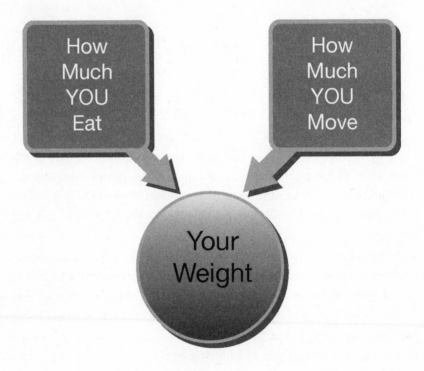

Your energy management system is an amazing system of checks and balances that can equalize weight over a wide range of conditions. Unfortunately, in modern life, our schedules and lifestyles do not allow it to do its job of increasing your activity or decreasing your caloric intake to maintain that balance. So that extra one hundred calories a day that come from one can of soda, one extra cookie, one afternoon candy bar, or one extra piece of pizza translates to an energy imbalance that, over a year, adds an additional five pounds of excess fat to our bellies. The insidious fat creep as a result of our obesegenic world is here to stay. Over two-thirds of us are currently the struggling casualties, with more on the way. Many are continually looking for help.

Many people give weight-loss advice. Most think they are experts on diets. They have tried most diets and are always ready to tell you what works and what doesn't. What I have found is that almost everybody giving you advice is trying to get you to either eat less or exercise more. Some try to get you to focus solely on your diet, saying that energy-dense food cannot be overcome with exercise alone. They are right. But long-term weight loss cannot be maintained without increasing activity.

Some say that exercise is the key to long-term success, because although you may lose weight slowly, you have a better chance of keeping it off. They are right too. But the packed gym in January is empty by the Ides of March. Where have all the people gone?

If you do not lose significant weight on a diet or with exercise, chances are you will get discouraged and not continue long enough to discover whether it works for the long term. There is a very simple solution: create safe and effective weight loss by reducing your energy intake, thus creating results that are observable and self-motivating. Add in progressive movement as you feel better and have more energy, and find a balance over time between your eating and your movement that is sustainable for the rest of your life.

Let's look at each of the three in more detail.

1. Reduce the Energy You Put in Your Body

When the first humans roamed the earth, their bodies were designed for food that was nutrient-dense and energy-sparse. As a result, our whole energy management system is set up to store and conserve calories. Sugar outside of that occurring in nature had not yet been discovered and added to foods. Can you imagine a world without refined sugar?

Until fifty years ago, the only people who became obese were rich people who could afford to indulge in fatty meats and creamy sauces, and were pampered by their butlers. The food industry began to make cheaper, energy-rich food to address world hunger. It accomplished that goal; now there are more overweight people than there are people starving. The industry left out one important condition: make the food healthy. Nutritionally polluted food accounts for over 90 percent of every-day food items. The majority of food is processed, not whole. The lack of healthy food choices makes it more difficult to find good fuel for your body. This means you must be more mindful.

There are many ways to lose weight:

- **Count calories** by reading all labels and weighing food. This may seem laborious, but research shows that it can be helpful if you will take the time to learn and do it.

- **Visually reduce portions** by guessing or using a visual analog such as a smaller plate.

- **Use prepackaged foods** for a cost-effective, easy-to-use system that doesn't require knowledge of nutrition. It works!

- **Use a glycemic index** to keep your blood sugar and insulin under control. High insulin levels put you in a fat storage mode.

- **Use a combination** of the solutions listed above.

2. Increase Your Energy Expenditure

Activity is essential to long-term weight control and optimal health, but how can we make it a reality?

> After the age of 20, we lose a pound of muscle a year. Each pound burns 70 kcal/day. That means by the time we are 40 years old, we have lost approximately 1400 calories a day of energy expenditure.

As you can see, to offset the progressive loss of muscle, flexibility, and energy expenditure, we must be mindful and purposely active in order to avoid a negative trajectory of this key determinant of your health.

In the next chapters, I outline the habits of motion that will offset this natural progression. You will begin slowly with stretching and flexibility and start moving more at work and play. This avoids injury and allows you to add activity incrementally as you lose weight. Add in a scheduled time to walk and progress each week. Add a weight resistance program over time, once your cardiovascular and muscle strength and flexibility are better. Add interval training, a progressive variable intensity of effort with your workout, so your body does not have time to adapt, as you continue to improve your cardiovascular fitness.

In this way, you are increasing your energy expenditure as you lose weight. This will offset the decrease expenditure, as you become smaller and lose actual body mass. Once you lose extra fat, you'll be amazed how much lighter you feel, physically and mentally. One woman who lost over a hundred pounds remarked that she felt as if she'd lost the weight of an entire human being.

3. Balance Your Energy for Life

The beauty of this simple formula is that it really works for long-term, sustainable health. When you focus on lowering your energy intake (which studies confirm is the most effective way to lose weight), you can lose up to one to two pounds per week. When you see results quickly, you will become more confident and reinforce the positive feedback. You'll have more energy, your clothes will fit better, people will notice, and, by using some of the tools and strategies I am about to teach you, you won't be hungry. (Or if you are, you'll learn how to overcome it.)

In a relatively short time, you'll start moving more, and you will be intrinsically motivated, rather than pressured to do it. You will be less likely to hurt your back or knees, because you have less weight to have an impact on your joints.

Also, because you are moving more by starting to walk and becoming more active, your increase in activity will offset the decrease in resting energy expenditure, which is a result of losing some weight.

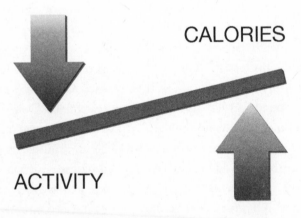

CALORIES

ACTIVITY

Once you have reached a healthy weight and waist circumference, you will have found a balance you can sustain for the rest of your life.

As you add higher levels of activity, such as weight resistance training, you will be able to eat more, as long as you maintain a balance.

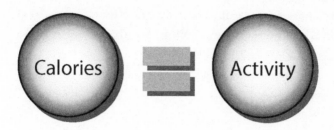

You can see how healthy eating and healthy motion are imperative
for reaching and maintaining a healthy weight, which is critical for
reaching optimal health. Two other important contributors to creating
long-term weight control and optimal health are quality sleep and the
ability to manage stress and create relaxation and a healthy mind.

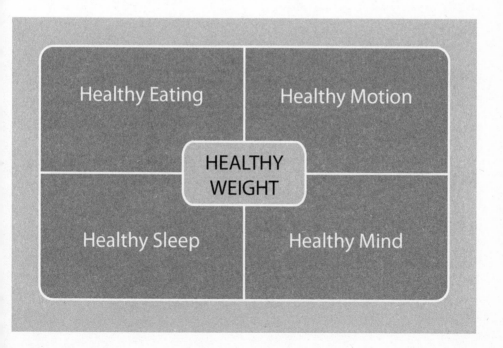

In the following chapters, I will specifically focus on each of these four critical habits of health to explain how each one is essential and synergistic to your health. Together we will progressively integrate and start your journey of mastering these foundations to create and maintain a healthy weight and optimal health.

CHAPTER 13

Discover the Habits of Healthy Eating

Tell me what you eat and I will tell
you what you are.[1]

—Anthelme Brillat-Savarin

MANY PEOPLE ARE CONFUSED ABOUT WHAT
healthy eating really means. There are *three fundamental desired outcomes* if you want to optimize your body and your health:

1. Match your caloric intake to your caloric outtake once you are at a healthy weight, to maintain your optimal weight.

2. Eat mostly foods that optimize your body's functions.

3. Avoid most foods that hurt your body's functions.

Seems simple, right? But I'm willing to bet you are not doing all three consistently. In my work, I find people who:

- Eat only organic whole food, but are thirty to forty pounds overweight.

- Are normal-weight but often consume high-glycemic, sugary foods.

- Avoid all red meat yet eat pasta frequently.

- Take every vitamin available, but don't eat fresh or frozen vegetables and fruits.

- Drink diet sodas with their double cheeseburger.

- Eat passively long after they are no longer hungry.

- Avoid breakfast, thinking they are saving calories.

- Think that if they are heavy they burn fewer calories than a much thinner individual.

The reality is that most of us do not fully understand what is best for us, which is why I am going spend time here to rectify that. I also want to be clear that I do not want you to adopt any habits of health strategies that you cannot live with forever. I am not going to pressure you into doing something you do not fully endorse.

First, *eat* to *live*; don't *live* to *eat*. If you are going to truly take control of your life, you must understand that your food choices can fuel a thriving life or lead it straight toward disease. Passive overeating (eating when you are no longer hungry) for comfort or pleasure or in reaction to emotion is a habit of disease that is feeding the wrong trajectory.

1. DESIRED OUTCOME: ENERGY IN EQUALS ENERGY OUT

To determine your starting point, what is the current status of your BMI and your waist circumference? High? Normal? Low?

In this section, we will focus on what you can do to lose weight by lowering your energy intake below your energy out if your current status is high. As you will find in the healthy motion chapter, you are limited in how much you can increase your energy expenditure to lose weight. It is especially important to focus on what you eat if you expect to lose weight.

Once you have reached your healthy weight as defined by your BMI and waist circumference, we will shift your focus to making healthy food choices while keeping your energy intake matching your energy out. Finally, in the last part of this section we will add some suggestions for those of you who are underweight.

Your Status: High Weight

Say you have a BMI of more than 24.9 and your waist is greater than 32 inches if you are female and greater than 37 inches if you are male. If you are currently overweight or obese, you need to lower your energy intake below your energy expenditure. There are two ways to drop caloric intake safely and effectively: the slower way and the faster way.

1. THE SLOWER WAY (A POUND OR SO A WEEK)

You can simply start lowering your caloric intake by cutting back your total calories and lowering your release of insulin and, thus, fat storage, which will decrease your cravings. This requires some preparation and knowledge of portion control and the glycemic index. The key skills here are portion control and understanding glycemic index.

Portion control. Either you can just reduce your portion sizes by 25 percent by estimating or you can use a visual analog and plate system. In the system I have developed, use a nine-inch plate and divide it into three sections. (I introduced this concept in my book *Dr. A's Habits of Health*; you can go to www.habitsofhealth.net to download the charts.)

Divide the food groups on the plate in these proportions:

- Fifty percent is fruit or vegetables, or about the amount of a medium-sized paperback.

- Twenty-five percent is starch, about the size of a tennis ball.

- Twenty-five percent is protein, about the size of a deck of cards.

An even easier, although not as effective way is to just cut your portion sizes of everything you eat by 25 percent. Cut meat into four pieces and put the fourth piece back on the serving plate. Place three rather than four squares of low-fat cheese on your plate.

Lowering the glycemic index. This is a way of categorizing foods by how high they raise your blood sugar and, as a result, your insulin level. By picking foods that are low glycemic and will not raise your blood sugar and your insulin you are helping your body remain healthy by keeping your body out of a fat storage mode, which will also help decrease your cravings for carbs. (I have created a color-coded system to make it easy to pick low-glycemic foods, which you can find in my book *Dr. A's Habits of Health*; you can download the charts at www.habitsofhealth.net.)

Understand that liquids contain significant calories and can result in empty calories (non-nutritive) without filling you up. Pay attention to what you drink: sodas have 150 calories; orange juice, 115 calories; coffee with cream, 90 calories. A 12-ounce beer is 140 calories; a 6-ounce glass of wine is 125 calories. A better choice is to substitute water, Crystal Light, Kool-Aid, or club soda.

Eating three one-hundred-calorie fueling meals and three smaller meals every three hours using portion control and low-glycemic food is a great strategy. The following pages provide some sample fueling suggestions.

Eat breakfast every day and choose healthy foods such as yogurt, fruits, or whole-grain cereals. Other tips:

- Always fill your plate in the kitchen; never put serving bowls on the table. (Studies show if we have more, we eat more.)

- Eat slowly to give your body time to send back the signals that you are full.

- Don't eat passively, which is defined as continuing to eat once your body tells you it is full.

- Always drink water first, as 30 percent of the time we are thirsty.

- Eat foods filled with water, which are less energy dense.

- Manage salad bars by avoiding bacon, potato salad, and putting balsamic vinaigrette on the side.

Sample Fueling Breaks

Meal replacements make excellent fueling breaks and assure that you're getting a 100-calorie, low-glycemic, nutrient-dense healthy food source.

- Cheese and tomato. One portion (size of two AA batteries) of natural cheese such as cheddar or Monterey Jack with one sliced tomato.
- Endive and tuna salad. One endive leaf with one tablespoon tuna salad, prepared with hummus in place of mayonnaise. Mediterranean Delights makes delicious, organic, low-fat hummus in flavors like tomato basil, and low-glycemic endive makes a handy container for the tuna salad.
- 3 oz mixed nuts (a small handful)
- 10 almonds and celery stick
- 29 pistachios
- 12 cashews
- 20 peanuts
- 2 tbsp sesame seeds
- 4 Brazil nuts. Great for getting your selenium!
- ½ sliced apple with 3 walnuts
- ½ apple with 2 tsp natural peanut butter. Make sure it's all-natural peanut butter: just peanuts and salt.
- ½ cup fresh strawberries with 2 tbsp light whipped topping
- 1 cup fresh cherries
- 1 medium apple
- ½ cup blueberries (high glycemic)

or strawberries (lower glycemic) with a dollop of yogurt
- 1 orange
- 1 pear
- ½ peach with 2 tbsp yogurt
- 2 cups raspberries
- 30 raisins
- Fresh veggie mix. 1 cup broccoli, red pepper, cauliflower with 1 tbsp low-fat ranch dressing.
- 6 pieces basil, sliced tomato, and hummus. My wife Lori's creation: put a dab of hummus and tomato on top of a basil leaf—delightful!
- Herbal lentils and one tomato
- Celery sticks with 1 tbsp natural peanut butter
- 1 cup fresh spinach salad with olives
- ¼ cup egg salad with lettuce or endive
- Half small avocado
- Cauliflower (size of paperback)
- 1 cup tomato and cucumber soup
- ¼ cup guacamole. Combine avocado, tomato, lime juice, and hot pepper to taste.
- Basil, tomato, and hummus (1 tomato)
- Grilled portobello mushroom sprinkled with cheese
- 5 cherry tomatoes with one portion cheddar cheese (size of two AA batteries)
- ½ cup endive and cottage cheese spread. In a food processor or

Sample Fueling Breaks

blender, mix cottage cheese, red pepper, fresh parsley, chives, and chopped jalapeno. Spread on endive.

- Eggplant pizza slice. Sprinkle a slice of eggplant with oregano and roast. Melt cheese on top.
- 1 cup vegetarian chili
- ½ cup edamame (soybeans)
- Half red bell pepper dipped in 3 tbsp hummus
- ½ cup cucumber slices
- 1 large dill pickle
- 1 carambola (starfruit)
- 2 cups baby carrots
- 3 celery sticks with 1 tsp natural peanut butter
- ¼ cup hummus and avocado dip with 3 celery stalks
- 1 cup mashed lentils and tomatoes
- Vegetables and dip. Choose either ½ cup cucumber slices, 6 celery sticks, 6 slices red pepper, or ½ cup raw broccoli florets and dip into 2 oz fat-free, sugar-free ranch dressing.
- 1 cup bean and chickpea salad. Toss diced celery, green pepper, cooked red beans, cooked chickpeas, and fresh parsley together with low-calorie balsamic vinaigrette.
- ⅓ cup low-fat cottage cheese with 4 olives
- Yogurt with ¼ cup berries. Yoplait Light plain yogurt is a great choice.

- ½ cup cottage cheese and ½ medium tomato
- 1 Yoplait Light Smoothie
- ½ cup low-fat cottage cheese with 5 strawberries
- 1 serving of string cheese
- 3 oz frozen nonfat yogurt
- 1 square 70% or higher dark chocolate with 5 almonds
- 1 whole deviled egg. Cut a hard-boiled egg in half, mix the yolk with hummus, and fill the egg.
- 1 cup of soup (cream of tomato, cream of chicken, chicken noodle, or vegetable)
- 1 slice Wasa crispbread with 1 oz smoked salmon
- 1 slice whole-grain bread (such as Fiber for Life) with 2 oz fat-free turkey breast
- ½ cup couscous with celery sticks
- 4 slices Melba toast
- 1 slice Wasa crispbread and ½ sliced tomato

Once you've reached a healthy weight, you can add these to the list as well:

- 1 cup fresh mango
- 1 cup cantaloupe
- 1 medium banana
- 28 grapes

This list should help you get started on ideas for your own small meals. Remember, each one should be low glycemic and no higher than 100 calories.

2. THE FASTER WAY (ONE TO TWO POUNDS A WEEK)

Use meal replacements. They are cost-neutral, clinically proven, and a very effective and safe way to help you lose weight quickly. I have found them to be a real lifesaver, especially for people on the go. I have used them for over a decade and helped tens of thousands of people lose and maintain their weight with great results.

The meal replacements I have used come from Medifast, which has been the leader in meal replacements since its inception in 1980. The previous criticism seen in the medical literature of meal replacements was that although they were very effective at helping you lose weight, they did not teach you how to eat healthy or address your lifestyle.

I have addressed this criticism by combining them with a comprehensive program that teaches you how to eat healthy and, with the habits of health, learn a new healthy lifestyle. In addition, to create a health-focused community, I cofounded a health network of coaches called Take Shape For Life, who both live and teach the mind-set to optimal health I have been describing in this book. In addition, I have found the meal replacements to be extremely effective for daily fueling, even after you have reached a healthy weight.

Studies from Harvard and UCLA suggest that meal replacement may be helpful for long-term maintenance.[2] They are a great way to get started because you simply pick out what you want and eat every three hours. They have portion control built in, and they are low glycemic. That starts you in the right direction and gives you time to learn the skills of portion control and glycemic index as you are effectively losing weight. You eat a meal replacement every three hours, which can be shakes, protein bars, soups, eggs, chili, sloppy Joes, macaroni, and others in a whole assortment of flavors. The intelligence is built into the products, which have been specified to have an almost identical nutritional footprint.

I can only recommend Medifast meal replacements because I am familiar with them and have used them exclusively.

They have twenty-four vitamins and minerals, and balance low-glycemic carbohydrates and healthy protein, which comes from legumes, although you can specify milk protein, if desirable.

I recommend one, healthy, whole-food meal a day, to complement the five-meal replacements. We teach you to choose lean meat, fish, or poultry, and a green vegetable or salad. During this weight-loss phase you must avoid eating high-glycemic carbohydrates.

Called the Medifast 5:1™, it will kick you into a fat-burning state in about three days; and you can lose, on average, two to five pounds in the first two weeks. After that, you will lose one to two pounds a week, and you are preferentially burning that unhealthy fat around the middle that is creating all the problems. As you lose weight and become more confident (a period I call the teachable moment), you are ready and eager to learn all the habits of health.

I have now detailed the two ways I recommend to unload the excessive calories from your body. The time this will take depends on which strategy you use and how much you need to lose. If you are using the faster method, you will have to restrict some foods during the weight loss, but it will be well worth it. By the time you reach your healthy weight, you will have learned the skills and strategies, and have the tools to eat a full range of food. Healthy people occasionally eat ice cream, steak, and lobster with butter, but they do not do it every day.

Let's focus now on your dietary intake once you reach a healthy weight.

Your Status: Healthy Weight

Let's say you have a BMI of 20 to 24.9, a waist of less than 32 inches if you are female, and a waist of less than 37 inches if you are male. As a starting point, make sure you have incorporated all of the following into your daily choices moving forward:

- Eat breakfast every day.

- Eat something every three hours.

- Use portion control.

- Eat mostly low-glycemic food.

- Eat lots of fresh fruits and vegetables.

- Approximately 50 percent of your intake should come from low-glycemic carbohydrates.

- Approximately 25 percent should come from healthy, lean proteins.

- Approximately 25 percent should come from healthy fats.

- Eat to satisfy your hunger.

Statistics demonstrate that as you become intentionally thinner, your risk for disease and death goes down. It is a major key in living a longer, healthier life:

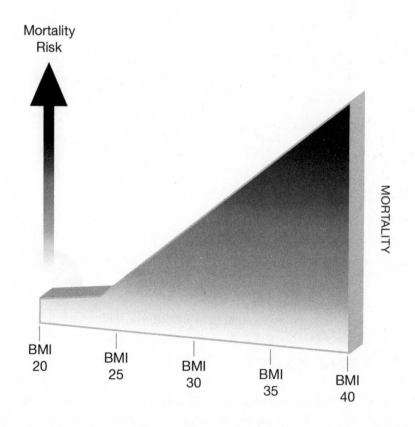

The ability to manage and maintain a healthy weight starts by finding your *set point*, which is the amount of calories you can consume per day to remain at your healthy weight. If you have been at a healthy weight, you will want to become even more observant as your energy expenditure goes down as you age.

If you are just reaching your healthy weight, you will have to adjust to find your new balance point. You will have lost some caloric expenditure with the weight loss because you have lost mass. Hopefully, you have been making progress in your activity, as I will outline next.

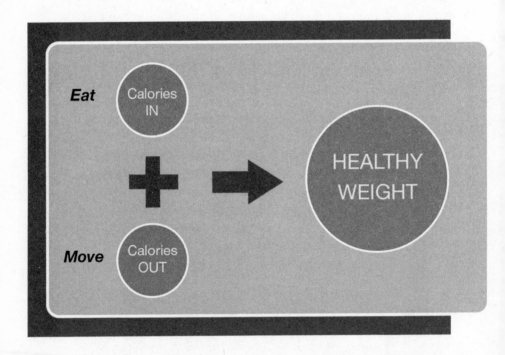

You did not get overweight in a day, and you will not totally master your weight control in a day. And if you have lost your weight quickly, you will want to keep pace and make sure you are learning the habits of health, especially the key ones in these four chapters.

As you master the habits of healthy motion and your caloric expenditure goes up, you will be able to eat more as your set point rises. A key relationship to master is that between hunger and fullness.

SATIETY: THE SCIENCE OF FULLNESS

The trick to maintaining a healthy weight is to eat enough healthy foods to satisfy both your physical satisfaction and your taste satisfaction and not more than your current set point allows. Research shows that we eat about the same volume or weight of food every day. So you want to get in the habit of eating lots of foods that are low in density (lots of water content) and have lots of volume (a large amount of food per calorie).

First, look at this list of healthy foods, filled with vitamins and minerals, that you can eat all the time:

HEALTHY SNACKS

This is a list of healthy foods filled with vitamins and minerals, which you can eat all the time because they have few calories and lots of volume:

Artichokes	Carrots	Parsley
Asparagus	Cauliflower	Radishes
Bamboo Shoots	Celery	Spinach
Beets	Cucumber	Squash
Bok Choy	Eggplant	Tomatoes
Bell peppers	Kale	Water Chestnuts
Broccoli	Lettuce (All Varieties)	Zucchini
Brussels sprouts	Mushrooms	
Cabbage	Onions	

Second, if you choose from low- and lowest-energy density (ED) foods, you will be balancing a full range of tastes, flavors, and textures, which creates fullness. See this chart about energy density:

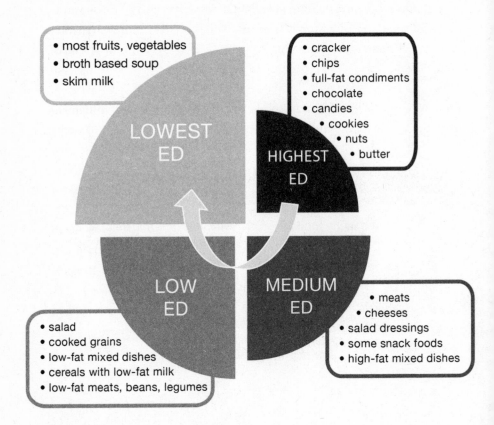

- most fruits, vegetables
- broth based soup
- skim milk

LOWEST ED

- cracker
- chips
- full-fat condiments
- chocolate
- candies
  - cookies
    - nuts
  - butter

HIGHEST ED

LOW ED

- salad
- cooked grains
- low-fat mixed dishes
- cereals with low-fat milk
- low-fat meats, beans, legumes

MEDIUM ED

- meats
  - cheeses
- salad dressings
- some snack foods
- high-fat mixed dishes

And because they have lower caloric values, you are creating fullness and maintaining a healthy weight.

Third, use macronutrients, the fuels your body runs on, to help balance your fullness and caloric ingestion. These are the three calorie producing categories of substances that make up your fuel choices.

As you can see, protein is the most filling and has less than half the calories per gram as fat, which is the least filling:

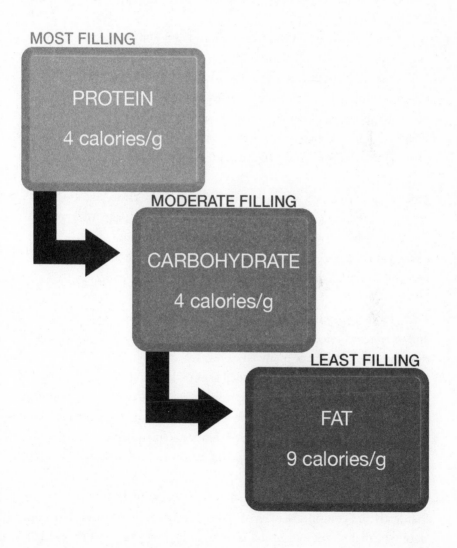

MOST FILLING

PROTEIN

4 calories/g

MODERATE FILLING

CARBOHYDRATE

4 calories/g

LEAST FILLING

FAT

9 calories/g

Alcohol is technically a macronutrient, but has no nutritive value. It may be considered an anti-satiety agent. Once your brain has been bathed in alcohol, the normal inhibitory areas become ineffective and your appetite, desire, and rationale all act against your best intentions and secondary choices. Why do you think the waiter first asks you if you would like a cocktail? Once you have your first drink, he's got you! It's like bait.

You rationalize that you worked hard today and you deserve it; then you proceed to eat everything that is not nailed down. *Order first*, then enjoy that cocktail if you are so inclined. Ask the server to remove the bread and bring water instead. Don't just leave the bread on the table. Remove the temptation completely. If you want an appetizer, order crab, shrimp, or grilled chicken on a stick, because the protein will help you fill up (just hold the sauce and use a little lemon).

Fourth, drink lots of water. Thirty percent of the time you are likely thirsty and not hungry. There are many other liquids (sugar-free) you can drink that also satisfy taste and break up the mundane taste of water: Crystal Light, Kool-Aid, iced tea, black coffee, club soda (great with lime), and diet sodas (occasionally). Or you can eat Jell-O pops.

Fifth, be very mindful and avoid those ingredients that creep into foods and have lots of calories. Peanut butter, butter, margarine, salad dressings, dips, and sauces all have many fat calories.

You can double your salad's total calories by using a regular dressing. Use spray-on, low-calorie dressings or at least have the dressing on the side. Dip your fork in the dressing and then pick up some greens. This could save you around three hundred calories. Remember that a reduction of one hundred extra calories a day can help you lose up to five pounds a year.

In the weight loss phase, you may have had to make some decisions that restricted your intake of what you wanted to remain in a fat-burning state. But that restrictive period is only in the first phase, when you are losing weight. The healthy weight phase is all about creating a balance of things you can do for the rest of your life. You are now making many small, seemingly insignificant decisions that add up.

Experiment with all kinds of different tastes and preparations. As I mentioned earlier, your taste satisfaction comes from the first three bites (95 percent), so if you crave a certain taste, eat high-volume, low-energy density foods first, which will satisfy your hunger. Then have a smaller piece of the forbidden fruit.

For example, I usually avoid eating bread at restaurants when I travel and lecture across the country. Sometimes I order a salad and appetizer for dinner, or share a meal with my wife Lori, in my normal routine. When I am in New York City (about four times a year), I immediately have Italian bread with butter because it is the best in the world, other than in Italy. (In Italy I have it every night! I have been there once.) I am very mindful in these special situations; because I know that if I deny myself that treat, I will not be satisfied with the meal. It is okay to treat yourself or continue to sample from the buffet that modern life offers us. As long as you respect the calories and limit the exposure, your body can overcome these moments of simply being human. After a meal like that, I'll walk the streets of New York or Roma for the next two days to help offset that heavenly bread.

Remember, with your new orientation toward health as a priority, you can now make these decisions because they support your radiant health.

Your Status: Low Weight

Let's say you have a BMI of less than 20. Most studies show that mortality actually starts going up once your BMI falls below 20, probably because people who have diseases were included in the studies. That is why I separate intentional weight loss from weight loss that is a result of disease.

I recommend that you use your belly fat and total body fat to determine if you have lost enough weight. Once your BMI is in the low 20s and your belly fat is gone, you have gained the health benefits. You could continue losing weight for vanity reasons. But since you want to achieve optimal health, I would not recommend going below 20 intentionally. And if you are a little older, it is always nice to have a few pounds as a buffer. If you're *unintentionally* losing weight, your next stop is your doctor for evaluation.

If you are trying to gain weight, the easiest way is through an increase of healthy fats such as fish, olive oils, complex carbohydrates, and proteins like nuts, which are very energy dense.

2. EAT MOSTLY FOODS THAT OPTIMIZE YOUR BODY'S FUNCTIONS

Being mindful can keep you focused on making healthy choices that will manage your calories and, at the same time, fuel your body with high-octane fuel. Start thinking of your body as if it were a Porsche, which you would never fill with regular gas (even in this economy). Your body is a far more magnificent, complex machine than a Porsche, and deserves to be fueled with the right energy.

Fruits and Vegetables Are Your Friends

Many people simply don't like fruits and vegetables. Yet both contain many helpful components to strengthen and protect; they are a key habit of health. You should eat a least five servings every day. They'll help control your weight while they optimize your health. Note: If you are using the 5:1 you will want to wait until you transition to healthy eating for life before adding fruit.

Keep fresh fruits like apples, bananas, or berries in bowls in the kitchen and dining room and, of course, plainly visible in the refrigerator. Instead of Oreos or chips, you'll reach for the healthy option.

Buy fresh frozen fruit and use it to spice up cereals and other breakfast meals such as pancakes and waffles, or yogurt.

Instead of soda, an obvious negative choice, have a can of 100 percent fruit juice (without high-fructose corn syrup) or a can of tomato juice. Keep these juices on hand, and eliminate sugary options.

Freeze bananas, strawberries, or grapes to make a yummy dessert instead of reaching for chocolate or cookies. Be mindful of your triggers and cravings, and carry packs of raisins, mandarin oranges, and other snack packs with you at all times.

Get packages of precut raw carrots and celery to snack on during the day.

When you must dine out with friends or clients, think about ordering soups, mixed vegetables, or a healthy salad with dressing on the side.

Put all kinds of vegetables on your wraps or sandwiches. Load salads with lots of vegetables and add as many bright colors as possible.

ADD FIBER

Fiber is another consumable that you should make sure you are adding to your diet. Fiber can help fill you up, lower your cholesterol and blood sugar, and improve intestinal health. Plant fiber comes in two forms:

Insoluble fiber does not dissolve in water and is not digested or absorbed by the body. Because it is filling, it reduces hunger. It also keeps the gastrointestinal tract clean and aids in regular bowel movements by pulling water into the colon. Good sources are brown rice, whole-wheat bread, cereals, seeds, fruit skins, vegetables, and my favorite—legumes.

Soluble fiber slows the breakdown of complex carbohydrates and helps reduce blood sugar. It dissolves in water, forming a gel-like mass that binds cholesterol in the stool. If you take enough, it can actually help lower your blood cholesterol. Some good sources are vegetables, legumes, fruits, and grains such as rye, barley, and oats. Each of these sources has about 3 grams of fiber per cup. Men need at least 38 grams a day; and women, 25 grams or more a day. My rule is that you should eat at least 20 grams of fiber per thousand calories, which is easily accomplished if 50 percent of your plate is fruits and vegetables. Supplement with bulk agents such as methylcellulose (Citrucel), guar gum (Benefiber), or psyllium (Konsyl). (Just make sure they are sugar-free.)

FISH OILS

I also recommend eating fish at least three days a week unless you are pregnant (due to the risk of mercury and other heavy metals effect on the fetus). Fatty cold-water fish are rich in omega-3 and other healthy phospholipids. It has numerous health benefits, including benefits to the immune system, brain, and heart. Also, the DHA in fish protects the brain and retina as well.

FRESH FISH

- Atlantic and Pacific Salmon
- Smoked Salmon
- Mackerel
- Bluefin Tuna
- Oysters and Squid

CANNED FISH

- Salmon
- Sardines
- Mackerel
- Tuna (in water, canola, olive oil, brine, or tomato sauce)

While eating fish regularly is a great way to stay healthy, given the diminishing supply of fish worldwide, you can supplement with one to two grams of pharmaceutical-grade (purity is a must) fish oil. Cold-water sources are the best (I would be happy to recommend one if you contact me).

BIOFLAVONOIDS

These powerful antioxidants, especially quercetin, found in apples, onions, broccoli, and tea, protect blood vessels from the harm of LDL cholesterol (bad). Pycnogenol, found in grape-seed extract, helps boost the immune system and strengthen the elastic recoil of your blood vessels.

3. AVOID FOODS THAT HURT
YOUR BODY'S FUNCTIONS

Most of us know to avoid fried food, fatty food (especially animal saturated fat), and refined sugar and white starches. Here is a list of foods to avoid:

- French fries

- Onion rings

- Fruit juices (unless pure fruit; most are only high-fructose corn syrup)

- Hot dogs

- Hamburgers (eat bison burger instead)

- Doughnuts

- White rice

- Sodas

- Cookies

- Candy

- Coconut or sunflower oils

- Other hydrogenated oils

- All trans fats

Avoid high-glycemic foods as much as possible. (Download the charts from www.habitsofhealth.net or review in *Dr. A's Habits of Health*.)

Cook with canola oil and use olive oil, but remember that a tablespoon is 120 calories.

When you use the barbecue grill, don't char your favorite meats and poultries. This forms substances called advanced glycation end products (AGEs). These extremely dangerous substances make your food up to two hundred times more immunoreactive, creating dangerous carcinogens and radicals that your immune system see as attacking your body with a vengeance. So you can use the barbecue to remove some of the unhealthy animal fat from meats, but do not let the meat or fat get a black charcoal-like appearance.

• • •

You are well on your way to understanding the habits of healthy eating. You now have new daily choices to use as alternatives and move up the path to improving health.

This would be a good time to create a structural tension chart of your desired goals for reaching a healthy weight and also your initial steps to eating healthier. Refer back to chapter 11 if you need some help in setting up your chart.

Let's now switch our focus to Habits of Healthy Motion.

CHAPTER 14

Discover the Habits of Healthy Motion

A man's health can be judged by
which he takes two at a time—
pills or stairs.[1]

—Joan Welsh

THE OTHER SIDE OF THE ENERGY EQUATION
is the energy you expend to operate and move your body. Some
of this expenditure is fixed, and some of it can be increased. Understanding this is important if you want to live in optimal health.

By improving the quality of your food, you enhance the thermic
effect of food and build mitochondria, the little power plants of your
cells, which improve energy utilization by increasing your movement.
Increasing your activity level with exercise is the ultimate, though not
immediate, goal, unless of course you already are on an exercise program.
It's important to integrate movement into your life gradually, through a
plan that is tailored to your current health, activity level, and weight. The
ultimate goal is to be actively exercising for thirty minutes, seven days a
week. That helps you create long-term optimal health, which is sustainable over decades, without taking too much time from our busy lives.

Thirty minutes a day for a lifetime of great health is a good invest-
ment. Yet most of us do not like to exercise. In fact, some of us might
absolutely despise it and find lots of great excuses to avoid it, ranging

from a lack of time, guilt for taking time away from the family, or the common one—gyms are intimidating, inconvenient, expensive, and make you self-conscious.

Overcome these excuses by focusing your life on the habits of health versus the habits of disease. Now that you have health at the center of your life and have removed the mental limitations, there's nothing standing in your way. You've got plenty of time. And you can do all of the things by yourself at home. (So much for having to wrestle with your self-image in a gym.) An inexpensive pedometer, a rubber mat, an exercise ball, a couple of water bottles for light free weights, and a pair of walking shoes are all you need to get started. Focus on moving your body more each day.

Movement is different from exercise. Movement happens every minute. You're always moving, in some way. But exercise is different. I define exercise as a designated time to intentionally work on your physical health through active movement. My goal is to intrinsically motivate you to schedule that thirty minutes for yourself. Then you endorse it rather than feeling that you ought to do something or you are being pressured by your peers or family.

There are two general areas that will help you optimize your habits of motion.

First, increase your total caloric expenditure, which will help you hold your set point even as you are losing weight. Remember, as you are losing weight, your energy expenditure will go down because you are losing some mass, which consumes calories. Your optimal health mind-set will continually center on a progressive increase in movement. So, unlike those who go on a diet, you will be making the necessary adjustments to offset that energy drop. And if you are already at a healthy weight, then you will be using the increase in caloric expenditure to get even leaner and also increase your energy intake.

Second, increase your cardiovascular endurance and your musculo-skeletal strength. You will add this when you are ready, in baby steps.

In a progressive fashion you should schedule time to work on both, as you feel comfortable and move toward a healthy weight. So I will review some physiology.

Your total energy expenditure (TEE) is made up of three components:

- **Basal metabolic rate** (BMR) makes up 60 to 75 percent of the total and is the energy used for general body functions.

- **Physical activity level** (PAL) makes up 25 to 30 percent and is the energy used when you move, walk, exercise, go to the store, or even pick up your mail.

- **Thermic effect of food** (TEF) makes up 10 to 15 percent and is the energy used to process and digest food. (In essence by adding high-quality protein, which I discussed in the healthy-eating chapter, you can slightly increase the energy required for digestion).

You can calculate your total energy expenditure using a very simple formula:

Your current weight (in pounds) x 11 kilocalories = TEE, if you are inactive. A calorie is the equivalent of 1 kcal.

Multiply your TEE by your activity factor (AF):
1.1 Inactive
1.2 for light activity
1.5 for moderate exercise
1.7 for heavy exercise

As an example: 162 lbs. x 11 kcal/lb. = 1,782 kcal x 1.2 = 2,138 kcal/day. (1 calorie =1 kcal)

This means that a normal-weight male could consume up to 2,138 calories of food a day and maintain his current weight.

Calculate your current TEE with your current activity level:

Step 1:

Your baseline TEE = _____ your weight (lbs.)

x 11 kcal/lb. = _____

Step 2:

_____ Your baseline TEE

x _____ activity factor = _____

Now you have a good idea of your current set point. This determines the amount of calories you can now eat and maintain your current weight.

For the rest of the chapter, I will add ways to increase your daily caloric expenditure, which will allow you to get even leaner, if that is your goal, or slowly increase your energy intake.

Now you can start burning more calories and move closer to your optimal health goals. There are two main ways to increase your energy expenditure. First, you can move more; second, you can add muscle mass.

I divide activity into two major categories:

- **General activity**—everyday movements at work and leisure when you are not intentionally trying to improve your health.

- **Scheduled exercise**—a specific time you devote to increased movement and weight resistance training with the specific goal of improving your health (not working or doing chores).

Let's say you are involved in working out three times a week, and your workout takes an hour. That is three hours of intense energy expenditure.

You have 168 hours (the number of hours in a week) in which to focus on small, incremental increases in energy expenditure in all 168 hours, even while you sleep.

If you are already in an active exercise program, read on, you may find some interesting ways to increase your caloric expenditure in everyday life.

1. GENERAL ACTIVITY

Let's put your mindfulness to immediate use. Humans were designed to conserve energy. If we are not mindful, we will always take the easy way. It's our nature.

For example, I was recently on a transcontinental flight and arrived in San Diego after six hours in a cramped seat. As I deplaned at 11 p.m., I was shocked to see a line of people waiting to get on the people mover. I just shook my head, stretched as I walked; once again the blood flowed to my brain and legs on the one-hundred-yard trek to the baggage claim. People are wired for comfort. Most take the easy path, unaware that they are missing endless chances to make the small, positive choices that build health.

But not you! You have the mind-set for optimal health.

Please read the following before you start increasing your activity:

Before you increase your activity and start actively increasing your energy expenditure, you should visit your physician for an evaluation.

Let him or her know that you are now focused on reaching and maintaining optimal health. Make sure your doctor is aware of your master plan so he or she can advise you of any special precautions to take.

Non-Exercise Activity Thermogenesis (NEAT)

One way to increase calories is through passive movement, or incorporating more movement into your normal day. Non-exercise activity thermogenesis (NEAT) refers to the energy you expend when you do trivial physical activities throughout your day, such as yard work, walking upstairs, or daily work-related activities.

Dr. James A. Levine at Mayo Clinic has extensively studied NEAT.[2] I introduce it as a comprehensive system to help expend calories in everyday activity in *Dr. A's Habits of Health*. It involves any time during the day when you are using your muscles and burning calories. Farmers or construction workers, for instance, are generally fitter than desk workers because their NEAT is higher. Increase your nonexercise activities throughout your day to increase your metabolic rate.

Start walking every chance you can. Buy a pedometer and spend the first couple of days making sure you know how to operate it and record your baseline steps per day. An average middle-age person walks between five thousand and six thousand steps a day, which decreases as he gets older. Most people over sixty have lowered their total steps to fewer than forty-five hundred a day, which is heading them straight toward disease.

Record your average daily steps: _____

The goal is to increase to ten thousand steps a day over the next several months. This is what is considered necessary to be healthy. You will get part of this from NEAT, starting today, and work up to a walking program when you are ready. There are several ways to work more steps into your daily life:

- Park far away from your destination in parking lots.

- Return your shopping carts to the storage racks.

- Walk in indoor malls in bad weather.

- Go to an art or history museum in bad weather.

- Go to the zoo.

- Work in your garden.

- Just say no to escalators and elevators.

- Do not drive, but walk to the local mailbox.

- Make several trips carrying your packages or groceries.

- Take the dog for a walk.

- Take your kids for a walk.

- Go for a hike.

- Take a walk in your local park.

- At your kids' sporting events, walk around the field while watching the game.

- Get a headset and walk around your office while on the phone.

- If you must watch TV, get up and walk around during commercials (not to the kitchen).

- Use the restroom and water fountain on the other end of the building.

- Take your lunch to work and walk to a park with benches; bring some colleagues with you.

Write down other times you can walk during your work and leisure:

_____   _____

_____   _____

_____   _____

Just say no to machines. You have many opportunities to do things manually. Understand that anytime you can use your muscles, you are shaping the trajectory toward health. Whenever your muscles are contracting, you're increasing caloric burn.

Here are some ideas:

- Sit up straight at work.

- Stand rather than sit.

- Use stairs whenever possible.

- Listen to music and tap your foot.

- Use a manual pencil sharpener.

- Rake leaves, rather than using the leaf blower.

- Shovel the snow.

- Wash your dishes.

- Go out and throw a ball to the dog.

- Stand up and change channels instead of using the remote.

Decide every day to stay mindful and aware of the opportunities for manual labor. Keep a log of what you did today and some things you could do by hand, just as your great-grandfather did.

Make a list:

- Plan an active vacation.

- Take up some new sports.

- Go to a sporting event.

- _____

- _____

- _____

- _____

- _____

- _____

All these activities fit into your normal work or leisure time. They do not take up any more of your normal day. As a result, you have no excuses for not doing them. As a great start, they can add a few hundred more calories per day of energy expenditure. (For a comprehensive discussion of NEAT and EAT, see chapters 13 through 16 in *Dr. A's Habits of Health*.)

Now I shift the focus to scheduled time, when you are specifically going to work on exercise and movement to create optimal health.

2. SCHEDULED EXERCISE: EXERCISE ACTIVITY THERMOGENESIS (EAT)

Scheduled exercise is what most people think of if asked to define exercise. It is the scheduled time when you are purposely moving your muscles to increase your physical health, as opposed to NEAT, which is motion that simply happens when you move at work and play.

Again, if you have not already had a physical, schedule it and tell your physician what you are doing, especially if you are planning to increase to heavier activity and planned exercise.

Once you are intrinsically motivated to take the intentional step to active exercise, schedule it for a thirty-minute period in your day. Your body prefers routine, so schedule it at the same time every day if you can. If not, make it fit into your work or child-care schedule. Either way, just do it. Please don't schedule it in the evening because it may interfere with another important habit of health, sleep.

Your Exercise Program (EAT)

If you're already an active exerciser, increasing the energy or activity you're already doing may help you reach your fitness goals. If you're not exercising, start a walking program.

First, make sure you have some comfortable shoes and loose-fitting clothes that absorb moisture but also breathe, so you do not overheat. Have reflective tape on shoes and clothes if you will be out after dark, choose a safe route, and avoid, if possible, roads used by motor vehicles.

Go outdoors for fresh air and sunshine, which are motivators for working out. Consider forming or joining a walking group for support and accountability. Indoors is okay, too, if you have a treadmill. Listen to music or watch TV on the treadmill to reduce boredom. (I can't believe I'm advising you to watch television, but if it keeps you walking, it's a good thing. But don't watch something negative.)

Stretch after you walk or after you have warmed up to avoid injury to tissues that are not yet warmed up. (People incorrectly stretch muscles before warming up, which can cause injury!) Also please start slow if you have not walked a lot. You are building habits for a lifetime, so you are in no hurry. You do not want to injure yourself.

Suggested Routine to Start
Warm-up—5 minutes at a 1-mile-per-hour (mph) pace,
approx. 160 steps
At pace—10 minutes at 2 mph, approx. 665 steps
Cooldown—5 minutes at 1 mph, approx. 160 steps

Once you have finished, make sure you spend about five minutes stretching your hamstrings, back, and calves. This twenty-minute session of around a thousand steps (about half a mile) will consume approximately fifty calories, if your BMI is around thirty. It will consume fewer if you are lighter and more if you are heavier.

Advance this program at your own pace. A general goal is to increase by five minutes each week to a moderate pace (three to four miles per hour). Continue this until you are walking five days a week for thirty minutes. This is approximately twenty thousand steps a week, which translates to about ten miles a week. This will keep you in an optimal state and is something you can do for decades to come. Keeping a log can be helpful to track your progress. Note: This is in addition to the 10,000 steps you are taking each day in your nonexercise movement.

Use the chart below to calculate how many steps are required to burn 1 kcal at your current weight (BMI). Remember that two thousand steps is approximately one mile.

ENERGETIC STEP VALUE (ESV)		
	(steps required to burn 1 kcal)	
Body Mass Index BMI	ESV (Female)	ESV (Male)
18 – 24.9 Healthy	36 steps per kcal	28 steps per kcal
25 – 29.9 Overweight	30 steps per kcal	24 steps per kcal
30 – 34.9 Class I Obesity	24 steps per kcal	20 steps per kcal
35 – 39.9 Class II Obesity	18 steps per kcal	16 steps per kcal
Over 40 Class III Obesity	12 steps per kcal	11 steps per kcal

The chart at right lists some other activities to substitute for or combine with walking.

Swimming is the best exercise because it does not create impact and supports flexibility and joint health, so you can do it when you're one hundred and older. I am such an advocate of swimming that I built a small resistance pool in my house so I can practice this habit of health all winter.

Other activities to substitute or combine with walking include:

- Cycling
- Canoeing
- Inline skating
- Ice skating
- Rowing
- Snow skiing
- Water skiing
- Hiking
- Volleyball
- Yoga

3. WEIGHT RESISTANCE TRAINING

Once you are getting into shape and have regained a full range of motion and flexibility, you may be ready to add weight resistance training. As you add muscle, your body benefits in several ways. First, you increase your caloric expenditure directly while you are lifting the weights. Second, since you are adding muscle, you burn approximately fifty to seventy calories/pound per day even when not actively lifting. Third, you strengthen your cardiovascular system and, in particular, maintain healthy bones, muscles, and balance.

I have developed this routine with an exercise physiologist from Johns Hopkins University. The sessions work either your upper body and core or your lower body and core.

UPPER BODY RESISTANCE TRAINING

- Core (upper)
- Chest
- Latissimus dorsi (back)
- Shoulders
- Arms

LOWER BODY RESISTANCE TRAINING

- Core (lower)
- Thighs
- Gluteals
- Hamstrings
- Calves

(You can go to www.habitsofhealth.net to download detailed suggested exercises for each muscle group. Full-color demonstrations are also included in the comprehensive advanced training in *Dr. A's Habits of Health*.)

Your weekly routine will be two thirty-minute sessions each week, consisting of:

1. A five-minute warm-up.

2. Five repetitions of five selected movements (a total of ten minutes) followed by a rotation of five different exercises that work the same muscle groups.

3. A five-minute stretch of the muscles you've worked.

I'll break it down so you get a better picture of what you will be doing in each session.

WARM-UP: FIVE MINUTES

Prepare your body to work out with five minutes of slow to moderate movement that increases your cardiac output, carries blood to your muscles, lubricates your joints, and helps prevent injury.

WARM-UP: FIVE MINUTES

- Walk in place while swinging arms.
- Mentally walk through the resistance movements you'll be performing in your resistance rotation.
- If you are at a gym, use the cardio equipment at a moderate pace.

RESISTANCE ROTATION:
TWO ROTATIONS OF TEN MINUTES EACH

This will challenge your muscles to grow healthier through short, intense workouts that stimulate all your muscle fibers. It will strengthen your bones and build lean, efficient muscles.

CHOOSE A SET OF 5 EXERCISES (ONE ROTATION)

- Begin each with a slow, consistent contraction (eight seconds); hold in place just before lockout (four seconds); then relax the muscles as you slowly return to your starting position (eight seconds), for a total of twenty seconds per exercise.
- Immediately begin another repetition, for a total of five per exercise.
- Rest for twenty seconds before starting a new exercise.
- Follow with a second rotation using a different set of exercises that work the same muscles.

One exercise repetition: each twenty-second repetition consists of a contraction phase, a holding phase, and a relaxation phase.

Complete five repetitions for each separate exercise.

Contraction Phase
8 seconds

Hold
4 seconds

Relaxation Phase
8 seconds

STRETCHING: FIVE MINUTES

Stretch the muscle groups you have just worked to improve your flexibility, increase your range of motion, and prevent soreness by encouraging your muscles to recover.

Again, this is just to get you started. I use some of these exercises to help people develop cardiovascular and musculoskeletal fitness. (You can go to www.habitsofhealth.net to download the exercises.)

My system is designed to minimize the amount of time you spend on exercise. Can you spare thirty minutes a day to walk five days a week and strengthen your muscles and bones on the other two days? I think you know the answer to that question.

This would be a good time to create a structural tension chart to organize your action steps in increasing your habits of healthy motion.

Now let's move on to a habit of health that most think is a luxury—sleep.

CHAPTER 15

Discover the Habits of Healthy Sleep

A good laugh and a long sleep are
the best cures in the doctor's book.

—Irish proverb

UNFORTUNATELY, THE FIRST THING SACRIFICED in our modern world is sleep. Only in the last few years have science and medicine begun to understand that without enough high-quality sleep, our health and lives unravel. Poor sleep rivals poor diet and inactivity as a reason that 90 percent of us languish in a state of being non-sick or have already slid onto the path to disease.

As you will soon discover, the habits of health affect how well you sleep. As you make those small, incremental improvements, you should sleep better. First, are you currently getting enough quality sleep? Do you:

- Wake up tired in the morning?

- Need a nap in the afternoon?

- Fall asleep watching TV?

- Have trouble focusing on the job?

- Are you sleepy after lunch?

- Feel irritable and/or depressed most of the time?

- Feel like you are not getting anything done?

- Drink alcohol to get to sleep?

- Have difficulty falling asleep?

- Have difficulty staying asleep?

If some or many of these apply to you, this section will help you understand and hopefully improve this most important habit necessary for long-term optimal health.

There are direct correlations among your weight, activity, diet, and sleep.

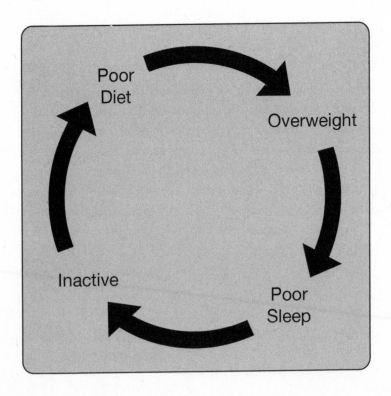

Lack of quality sleep affects the secretion of leptin, ghrelin, and cortisol, the hormones that regulate our weight. Leptin provides feedback on our current energy status. When we sleep well, the levels increase and we are not hungry. When we do not sleep well, the leptin secretion goes down. Studies have shown that when our leptin level goes down, the secretion of cortisol increases, which also increases appetite. And we crave high-energy foods, such as fat and sugars. That's why that stop at Dunkin' Donuts on the way to work in the morning for coffee and pastry is so desirable and so unhealthy.

The paradox of poor sleep is that we get heavier from eating unhealthy food and we are too tired to move as much. The extra weight also has a tendency to cause or aggravate obstructive airway breathing issues, which further decreases the quality of sleep, leading to more weight gain. Integrated health requires us to look at all the habits of health.

Let's address some basics for improving your sleep and health.

- How much sleep do you get? _____ Hours per night (from the time you fall asleep until the time you open your eyes in the morning is your sleep time minus any time you were awake during the night).

- What is the quality of your sleep?

- Do you sleep through the night without awakening?

- Do you wake up refreshed and ready to attack the day?

- Do you wake up on your own before the alarm clock?

- Do you never need medications or alcohol to induce sleep?

If you answered no to any of the above questions, you can probably improve the quality of your sleep.

DO YOU SNORE?

There are some very organic reasons why you may not be able to sleep. Modern sleep science is identifying many sleep breathing disorders that can affect the quality of your sleep. Most of these are vastly improved by practicing the habits of health, and reaching a healthy weight is particularly effective.

I recommend visiting a sleep doctor if you continue to snore or have poor quality sleep. A sleep doctor may be very helpful in helping you improve your sleep. Also simply sleeping on your side can be helpful, as you are getting healthier.

On average, people should have approximately six to eight hours of sleep. Recent studies, reversing earlier ones, say an average woman should have about twenty more minutes of sleep a night than a man.[1] We know that people who sleep less than six hours or sleep more than eight are at higher risk for disease. There are, of course, some people who need less or more hours of sleep. How about you? How many hours are you getting? The best way to figure out how many you need is to see what time you wake up naturally about halfway into your next vacation (not after a night of heavy partying).

If you do not get to bed, you have no chance of getting to sleep. Sleep is a critical habit of health, so make the decision to plan your schedule around the proper allowance for you.

HOW CAN I IMPROVE MY SLEEP?

Step 1: Are You Lark or an Owl?

Your melatonin level and core temperature determine the optimal time for your sleep. Figure out whether you function better in the evening or the morning and adjust your schedule if possible. Also, make sure you do not change your daily routine radically and try to catch up on weekends. Sleeping an additional two to three hours on weekends is like flying across time zones. Monday morning will come way too early.

Discipline yourself to wake up the same time every morning. If you need to catch up, take a five-minute nap during the day.

Step 2: Figure Out What Time to Get Up

Count back to determine your required sleep time (six to eight hours) and when to get up to include time to have a healthy breakfast. You can tweak this when you go on vacation. Your bedtime is when the lights are out, your head is on the pillow, and your eyes are shut. Schedule sleep! You will know you have gotten it right when you wake up in the morning before the alarm goes off.

Step 3: Plan Your Day and Evening

Many daily choices either set you up for a great night of sleep or not. What can you do during your day or evening to help create healthy sleep?

DURING THE DAY

Once you wake up, get out of bed. No snooze alarm for you! The bed is for sleeping and lovemaking (I highly recommend more of both as habits of health). Get out in the bright sunlight as soon as possible. Sunlight is critical to promoting a state of wakefulness, especially in the morning and afternoon. Your eyes sense the bright light and lower your melatonin levels, thus increasing your wakefulness.

Take your sunglasses off for a period of time and soak in the sunlight. If during the day, you start feeling sleepy, go for a five-minute walk, rather than grabbing a coffee.

NOTE:

Caffeine has a half-life of six hours, which means that if you have an afternoon coffee to get through the day, when you want to go to sleep at 11 p.m., you will still have caffeine swirling in your brain. It blocks the receptors necessary for falling asleep.

Start increasing your NEAT and EAT activities to increase your core temperature. The more awake you are during the day through activity and sunshine, the easier it will be to turn off at night.

You do not have to give up coffee or caffeinated tea; just savor them in the morning. Once noon rolls around, limit or avoid anything caffeinated and make sure you have nothing with caffeine in it within three hours of sleep time.

Avoid eating a large meal within three hours of retiring. If you really need something, have a small glass of skim milk, chamomile tea, or a small snack (low fat, low glycemic, low calories). For optimal sleep, eliminate high-glycemic foods throughout the day and avoid energy-dense or fatty meals in the evening. A small fueling or meal replacement is okay.

IN THE EVENING

Your time away from work is very important for your mind, which I will discuss in the next chapter. It is equally important for an optimal night's sleep. On your way home, make a mental note of any tasks or activities that you need to do. You should do anything that requires strenuous activity or time for EAT exercise at least two hours, and preferably more, before bed.

Here are some guidelines to help you prepare for what I call sleepy time:

Review your day. Pay attention to all the things you did during the day. The more activity, more sunlight, less caffeine, and better the food, the easier it is to turn on the sleep factors.

Decrease stimulation. You were designed to be awake during the day. Our ancestors went to bed when the sun went down and the campfire burned low. Lower the lights in the evening to turn off your pineal gland; called the third eye, it is a light sensitive endocrine gland in your brain that is responsible for regulating your state of alertness. It does this by cooling you down and increasing your release of melatonin, which induces sleep. Turn off anything with an on button at least thirty minutes before you plan to hit the pillow.

Minimize liquid ingestion and avoid any liquids two hours before bed. Empty your bladder just before turning in. Avoid activity so you can properly cool down and increase your melatonin production. If you have pain or allergies and are on medications, take those an hour before bed. Pain or upper airway blockage can interrupt sleep.

Avoid alcohol within ninety minutes of bedtime or have none at all, if you are having difficulty in falling asleep. Alcohol is a stimulant and then a depressant and may induce sleep, but it actually decreases the quality of sleep.

Resolve all family or other issues before getting ready for bed. We have a rule in our family: never go to bed mad.

I think of this as calm time. You should actually develop a ritual, which is a special time to prepare yourself for sleep. Help family members develop their own routine so that they all are in alignment. Introduce these ideas as soon as possible to your routine and home.

Make your bedroom visibly calming, mentally relaxing, and free of any stress and clutter. Put your children, dogs, cats, and other critters in their own beds.

If your partner snores or has restless legs, get him or her to the doctor as soon as possible.

Take a nice warm shower or bath, which will warm you up. Then the cooldown will simulate your core temperature dropping and release melatonin, helping to induce sleep.

Wear comfortable, cool clothes so you do not overheat.

Mentally let everything go.

THE ULTIMATE SLEEP CHAMBER

- Color can induce sleep. Pick comfortable, soothing colors.
- Lights should be on dimmers and at least an hour before put them at a low setting.
- Scented candles are fine as long as you blow them out when you get in bed.
- Completely darken your room. Put black tape over any LED lights in your room. Use blackout curtains or blinds.
- Get the TV out of the bedroom.
- Put a drop of scent such as chamomile, jasmine, lavender, or sandalwood in your bath or on your pillow case.
- Make sure your mattress firmness is right for you and has a dampering system so if your partner moves, you do not feel it.
- Regulate the temperature of the room so it is neither too hot nor cool.
- Keep the room cool so your core will be cool.
- Do not use artificial heat generators such as heating pads or electric blankets.
- Infrared quilts and sheets self-regulate and keep your body temperature neutral.
- Maintain adequate ventilation.
- Remove all clutter so the room is relaxing.

Make healthy sleeping a priority and I suggest you create a structural tension chart to help guide your new healthy action steps to choices that will improve your sleep.

Now, let's focus on probably the single most important factor in creating and maintaining your optimal health—a healthy mind.

CHAPTER 16

Discover the Habits of a Healthy Mind

The root of all health is in the brain. The trunk of it is in emotion. The branches and leaves are the body. The flower of health blooms when all parts work together.

—Kurdish saying

THE LEGENDARY GREEN BAY PACKER COACH Vince Lombardi started every new season with the basics. His famous line was, "Gentlemen, this is a football." The first time Lombardi espoused that now famous quote, his star athlete, all-pro Max McGee responded: "Uh, coach, could you slow down a little? You are going too fast for us."

This is your new season, one in which you have the opportunity to put your health at the center of your life by starting with the basics. This season can be a fresh new start.

But, unless you slow down enough to implement the simple daily choices that you must make, your life won't improve. You may believe in the theory of good health and understand how to practice the habits of health. If you truly desire health, then you need to understand that what you see, hear, and think about has a direct physiological effect on the body. The mastery of understanding is important, but even more important is optimizing the connection between your mind and your body, because it is the ultimate key to success. Now it's time to execute.

When I finished my training from one of the most prestigious training programs in critical care, I felt well equipped to care for even the sickest people. In the first few years of practice, I used numbers, blood work, pulmonary function tests, and cardiovascular parameters to determine if a patient could safely go through a life-threatening operation. Later on, I would review the numbers to understand the patient's risks and the best techniques for the preoperative period. But no matter how high the risk, I made the decision to proceed after a meeting with the patient in my office in the ICU.

I would sit next to the patient, look in his eyes and, with great empathy, ask him if he wanted to live. I would level with him and explain that we were about to get him through this aortic arch resection (or some other high-risk operation) and that I needed him fighting side-by-side with me. It would be a team effort.

If the patient looked at me and, without hesitation, said yes, that was enough for me. I knew we'd be a great team and that we'd probably have a good outcome. But if the patient didn't agree to fight with me, I knew the prognosis wasn't going to be as good.

Your mind is your greatest asset. In order to succeed at anything in life, you've got to be all in. The old way of thinking is gone. In the past, you let your circumstances dictate your emotions, your eating habits, and your responses to surroundings, but now everything is different. You are the dominant force in your life.

The way you think and choose will dictate your health path. You can respond with conscious choice to life's challenges, rather than overreact with negative thoughts that can derail your health and life. Instead of reacting with emotional eating, you can stop, hit pause, and think about your next step. Be kind to yourself. Stop judging. Be mindful. Your brain works for you, not the other way around.

At this point in your journey of discovery, you have all the skills you need to fully integrate your mind in optimal health. Despite that, there will be obstacles. Your body's physical design is in conflict with the modern world, and your mind is, too. Each day, you are bombarded with information and data. There are more than seventeen thousand different symbols and logos that saturate our senses daily. Being mindful can be a challenge.

As I discussed in chapter 10, there are two parts of your autonomic nervous system that run your internal processes. The sympathetic and parasympathetic systems control body functions such as breathing, heart rate, and your digestive system. Ten thousand years ago, the parasympathetic was the default mechanism, which would quiet the body to achieve a wonderful state of calm and alertness capable of being very mindful of our surroundings and any potential dangers.

In that very desirable state, the heart rate is slow, breathing is deep from the diaphragm, and the stress level is low. But, today, we operate at a much higher pace, connected to smartphones, computers, social media, and other electronic leashes. We operate in a high sympathetic tone, with shallow and faster breathing, alternating with breath holding and anxious feelings when someone doesn't respond to our text or e-mail. In this state, we are programmed to be upset if someone isn't instantly available. Add the television and the computer, and we have a dichotomy in which we are more connected globally, but more emotionally and relationally disconnected from those sitting next to us.

For example, I recently observed a family of four having dinner at a restaurant table next to us. Within five minutes, what might have been a wonderful opportunity to have some quality family time turned into four people, all somewhere else. Dad was on his cell phone, mom was on her iPad, the son played games on his phone, and the very young daughter played a Barbie game. When their food was served, they barely acknowledged each other and proceeded to wolf down their food and then were gone. Is this the kind of life we are all living? I couldn't help but notice that my own family and I were still deeply involved in our conversation and enjoying our time together over tea and sorbet. This kind of bonding takes intentionality. (Next time you are out to dinner with friends, build a cell stack in the center of the table with your cell phones. If anybody touches a phone during the dinner, he or she has to pay for everyone's dinner.)

Your healthy mind is dependent on your input through your associations and encounters and your own internal thought process. At the very center of your new mind-set to optimal health is how you focus on being mindful and kind. Being kind to yourself and others in small, seemingly insignificant daily choices will change the dynamics in your relationships. This is going to take time, because many people have become negative and have not become mindful. Focusing on the good, demonstrating kindness and empathy, and living in the moment can change you, those around you, your whole community, and even the world.

For example, on that fateful day, 9/11, when the United States was under a devastating terrorist attack, the country and even the world came together. For a month or so, we were kinder, more thoughtful, more unified, and collectively as humans in a higher state of awareness of our communities. Despite the horrific tragedy, we felt more connected and had a sense of social intelligence together.

You can create that for yourself; it actually is contagious. Try this. During your next conversation with someone, listen closely, stop the dialog in your own head, and just listen. Ask questions if you didn't understand something she said, but mainly just listen. Watch the effect it has on her facial tone, body language, and actual words.

We are in a world that has stopped listening; we are missing a lot all around us. Your child may have just made a discovery. A friend may need a few words of comfort and reassurance. Or it may be you are responding to an emotion that you didn't even realize you were feeling.

In this chapter, I am going to give you some new exercises and organize some discussed previously in the mindful and relaxation section. These ideas and skills will help you during those hundreds of daily moments, so you can make the adjustments necessary to improve the outcome of your health and life.

AWARE: INSIDE AND OUT

Start by training your mind to be aware of what is going on in the moment. This is the first essential to bring to your consciousness, the emotions you are feeling in the moment. It is a critical skill. Once you are aware of the emotion, you have the opportunity to control the outcome. This helps identify triggers, which lead to eating the wrong foods or saying the wrong things.

If you are in tune with your body, you will be able to pick up on your emotions. Anytime you feel that something isn't right (your breathing changes, your heart rate increases, or you get a bad feeling in the pit of the stomach), immediately stop, challenge, and choose:

STOP

Your mind and your body are tightly linked. The physical sensations, such as a gut feeling, are reminders. Be mindful to what's going on in your mind and body.

CHALLENGE

By getting good at stopping, you are putting yourself in a position to know how to control your response to a negative feeling or emotion. Being mindful allows you to stop and think about your response. Do I get up and walk to the refrigerator? Do I overeat? Should I pour myself a glass of wine?

Did you ever stop to think why you respond the way you do? Emotional triggers can drive eating and unhealthy choices. Be aware of them. For example, if you think you are not smart because you didn't finish school, and then someone says something that you think makes you look dumb, chances are you are going to react in one of the following ways:

- Lash out with anger and an aggressive response.

- Say nothing and then go and eat a bag of M&Ms.

- Go sign up for a course in calculus.

If, instead, you could stop and ask yourself: Do I really need to make sure that everything someone else says reinforces that I am smart? (or pretty, or artistic, or a great athlete?)

The most important thing you need to know about managing your mind-set involves carefully filtering your triggers and emotions. Work to eliminate toxic thoughts and limiting beliefs. If you think you are not smart, diplomas, smart awards, or Nobel prizes will never be enough. Make a decision to wake up each day renewed, full of hope, and focus on what matters most to you. Think first that, no matter how you feel, you are going to do what is necessary to create your desired outcomes. Being mindful of your mental and emotional health and thoughts also means recognizing what areas you are sensitive in. If you need to continually support your ego, you will be a pawn for others to control you, and your quest for optimal health is going to be difficult.

As a physician, I remind people that cultivating mental health is important to optimizing physical health, too. A negative mental outlook increases stress levels and affects the way your mind and body interact. So in those situations where you find yourself getting upset, ask yourself if what is happening is real or just a perceived or imagined threat. Is this something worth focusing on? When you put things into perspective, you stop worrying and obsessing about every little facet of life and what others think of you. This leads to contentment and freedom. Choose the thought or outcome that moves you forward.

CHOOSE

Take a deep breath or drink a glass of water and smile and move on to what really matters. Focus on letting go; do not internalize negative feelings of low self-worth that lead to the habits of disease. It is going to take practice, so here are some ways to break that cycle:

- Take a slow deep breath similar to a deep sigh and let the tension and anxiety leave with your exhale. Repeat until you feel a calmness return before acting.

- Stop thinking that your emotions are good or bad. They are feelings.

- You cannot control. Stop trying. Instead bring your emotions to instant awareness by sensing and recognizing what emotion you are feeling, and allow yourself time to process before acting.

- Recognize when you are under stress or in a difficult situation and become even more aware of your feelings and your responses.

- It's fine to feel a certain way. Learning how to manage that feeling is the important part.

- Keep a journal and figure out what pushes your buttons so you are prepared next time.

- Ask yourself if you get mad or angry and tell someone how it feels, does it make a difference?

- Ask yourself why you act that way. (Hint: Usually it's your ego.)

- Ask someone you trust to help you recognize and manage your emotions.

- Offer compassion and kindness even to those who are difficult; it is amazing how quickly kindness and cooperation can start the healing process.

MANAGE YOUR INSIDE AND OUTSIDE

The other part of managing your emotions and your surroundings is to be well rested. When we have not slept well, we are more likely to be in a bad mood and say and do things reactively, rather than rationally. So the habits of healthy sleeping need to be a priority for emotional management as well.

Other important ways to create a mental environment of mindfulness, self, and social management are:

- Take time off to recharge your batteries.

- Unplug daily. Find a quiet time when you disconnect from your electronic leash and do something that you enjoy. Listen to music, go for a walk, do ten minutes of stretching or yoga, or just take a five-minute nap.

- Take time on the weekends to recharge as well. Go to a museum with the kids; cozy up with your partner and build a fire.

- Plan time off from work; go on a vacation, maybe on a beach doing nothing or traveling to foreign country.

- Embrace activity, the habit of healthy motion.

- Embrace good food, the habit of healthy eating.

The core daily choices all work together to synergistically uncover a mind-set that will help you create optimal health. Now that you are in charge of your health and your life, you are ready to take over your inner thoughts. This cartoon will remind you:

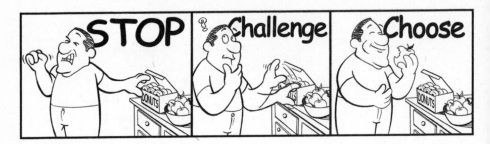

One area we hardly ever discuss is our internal conversation with ourselves. We have tens of thousands of thoughts per day, and the ones that are usually most prominent are the ones we talk to ourselves about. There is nothing wrong with self-talk, because it helps you get through your day and manage tasks. When I am packing for a trip or before I leave the house, I may catch myself saying, "Let's see, where are my keys? Did I blow out the candle? Do I have my phone?"

But when the self-talking becomes negative, it does not serve us. It actually gets in the way of rational thought and the ability to choose the habits of health.

First, you are the one responsible for your health and your thoughts. You need to be the dominant force in steering yourself toward the optimal health you desire. You are not blaming others for what you are in charge of accomplishing, so stop blaming yourself for other people's issues. You are responsible for you and they are responsible for them. And even though you certainly have a responsibility for integrating your children into society, they also have a responsibility to be responsible. As parents, we can be so hard on ourselves when our kids make bad choices. They are developing people and will not always do what we say.

Speaking of parenting, we have to learn to not say things to them that could affect how they think about themselves. We should never say they are stupid. Instead we should say something like, "maybe there was a better choice you could have made in that situation, so let's work together to make that choice." Again, you should never stereotype them as stupid; because of your position of influence, they may start believing it is true.

Second, if you never say your children are stupid, why would you call yourself stupid, or ugly, or a hundred other negative things? Stop judging yourself. Treat yourself with the same kindness and good intention you would your children, friends, and those you love.

If you make a mistake and eat that brownie, don't say that you have no willpower, but rather, you made a bad choice. Stop stereotyping yourself, and start making more choices that move you to your mind-set for optimal health.

The thought of failing can also create internal dialog: "It seems too difficult." "I am not sure I can do this." "It seems as I go forward that everything is stacked against me." "I have failed at everything I have ever done before. How could this be different?" If you get beyond the emotions, all those feelings of self-doubt, worry, and guilt are just that: feelings.

Now that you have the ability to separate your emotions from your responses, you can focus on your health and make progress. If you have a bad day or make an unhealthy choice, it will no longer derail you, but just give you an opportunity to build from the experience. Sometimes it is our failures that give us the best opportunity for growth.

I have had times when, after I failed, and I was more likely to do a critical evaluation of why I failed so that I could regroup and make another stab at it. Success actually has the potential to slow down our growth because we find ourselves distracted— celebrating and not learning. You really only fail if you give up, so always recalibrate to what you are working toward, and keep your emotions from being the centerpiece of your life.

Your focus, plan, and surrounding support can now overcome the ability of negative self-talk to sabotage your progress toward health. Your regrets from the past or your fear for the future have no ability to influence the only time that really matters: the present. By being fully present in the moment through mindfulness, you can make the next small choice that adds into the desired outcome, which is your optimal health.

In addition, focusing on the needs of others is a powerful neutralizer of negative thoughts. By being kind and feeling compassion, we become connected to each other and we feel better about ourselves as well.

Stress reduction needs to be a big part of our daily routine to take us out of that high sympathetic state and reestablish that parasympathetic, calm, relaxed state that is so critical. In chapter 10, I identified how stress affects you negatively and gave you some breathing and relaxation techniques. Use them at work and at leisure to adjust your thermostat to a more relaxed, mindful place. Learning to breathe deeply and meditate are great starting points in this process.

• • •

Here's a review of how you can take command of the daily chaos. Use this anytime you are feeling out of sorts, tired, overwhelmed, or bored, by breathing and creating a healthy state instantly:

- *Stop whatever you are doing, sense the speed and rate of your breath, and inhale.* Since your breathing is normally controlled by your autonomic nervous system (involuntary), what you will first do is *evaluate yourself.* Is your breath more rapid and shallow, which tells you it has been taken over by stress? *Recalibrate.*

- Don't allow your breathing to be involuntary. *Pull it into your voluntary nervous system by becoming aware* of how you are breathing.

- Now as you *wrestle away control, you can slow down your breathing.*

- You can then shift from the shallow upper-chest breathing to a deep breath from your diaphragm in which you *sense your belly expanding* more than your chest.

- This process *will calm, refocus, clarify your thoughts, and give you command and mindfulness in the present moment.* It allows you to become the dominant force in control over your body and to always reset it to a healthy state, despite what is happening around you.

Do this many times a day. I do! It is the habit of health! It will put you in charge of your health.

Now would be a good time to create a structural tension chart outlining the secondary choices you plan on making to help improve your emotional intelligence and reduce your stress levels.

A healthy mind is the gateway to discovering your optimal health. You now have the key foundational pieces to change your trajectory and live a longer healthier life.

Epilogue: Taking Back Your Life

> Health is a large word. It embraces not
> the body only, but the mind and spirit as
> well . . . and not today's pain or pleasure
> alone, but the whole being and outlook
> of a man.[1]
>
> —James H. West

THROUGHOUT THIS BOOK, I'VE COVERED THE importance of organizing your life around what matters most. Until now, I have been talking about how you can reduce the effect of stress, external hazards, and life's issues on your mind and body.

Now you have the stop-challenge-choose method to successfully manage perceived threats to your ego and to decrease the effect of these emotional stress creators on your body. I want to discuss ways, beyond just reacting to stress, to actually eliminate stress from your life and potentially put you in a much better position to optimize your total health.

Imagine if you could actually change your underlying structure to create a relatively stress-free environment. This is similar to removing the bad food from your pantry. To start this exercise ask yourself, have you organized your life around what is most important to you? Write down what is most important to you (these can be things you already have or desired outcomes):

_____   _____
_____   _____
_____   _____
_____   _____
_____   _____
_____   _____
_____   _____

The things we decide are most important to us can be generally categorized into extrinsic and intrinsic aspirations.

Extrinsic aspirations are material things, such as cars, houses, boats, and so on. Intrinsic aspirations are things inside, such as things we want to do, or sharing love, compassion, friendships, involvement, and fulfillment. Now, go back and review all those things that you listed above and put either an *E* or *I* beside each one.

Are most of your desired outcomes or things that you either
    have or want extrinsic or intrinsic? _____

Now here comes the tough question.

Are you currently fulfilled, happy, involved, and satisfied with your life? There are generally six categories of psychological needs that humans strive to fulfill. *First* is the desire to follow your own path and do things because they matter to you. Humans do not like being controlled. *Second* is the something that matters to you and that you want to become good at it and grow as a person. *Third* is the desire to feel relevant and leave a legacy, to relate with others in a fashion that brings great personal satisfaction. You can experience this by being a great parent, writing a great novel, helping your community, or starting a business. These intrinsic measures create self-motivation and bring involvement and fulfillment.

If these intrinsic needs are filled, they are sufficient, because they create a sense of well-being in your life. When you're in that state, your stress levels are much lower. The hassles of everyday life have less impact. Fulfillment changes your underlying structure and clears out those land mines that affect you when you are not happy or fulfilled.

The three categories of extrinsic psychological needs are those things that most of us grow up coveting:

- *First* is wealth or the ability to have enough money to buy whatever we want, which often can be more money.

- *Second* is fame, to be famous and sought after.

- *Third* is to be attractive so that people are attracted to you.

These three psychological needs create the need for many more variations. Having money is better than not having money. Being well-known can get you into restaurants; being attractive and having people drawn to you can be satisfying. But these three things don't create more satisfaction with life or optimal health, and eventually those who seek it end up wanting more. And the desire for more creates more stress, which is the opposite of optimal health.

So, if the activities you are currently doing each day don't satisfy your intrinsic needs, maybe it's time to do a life assessment.

YOUR OCCUPATION

Are you satisfied with your current position? _____

If not, are you in control of the ability to change it? _____

Is your position stressful? _____

If your occupation is satisfying, congratulations! You're a rare individual. Few people are actually happy in what they do. If not, can you advance, change, or leave to find a position that you are more intrinsically motivated by?

When I coach individuals, sometimes I find that the stress in their work lives comes from poor communication. If you can communicate your frustrations and concerns or better understand what is expected, it can go a long way toward reducing stress. Or, it might be time to go in a different direction. Changing careers can be scary, but maybe the biggest regret would be to do nothing and continue in an environment that is robbing you of your health.

After I had trained as a critical care physician, I set off in my early thirties to help cure the world. I worked long, hard hours, enjoyed the challenge. Since I was single, it really didn't matter that I had this crazy schedule. I made great money, lived in a neat condo, took amazing vacations (although not often enough), and was totally intrinsically motivated. Then I met Lori, the love of my life, and shortly after, we had two wonderful daughters, first, Savannah, and then, Erica.

Shortly after Savannah was born, I noticed that the long hours seemed to bother me more. I would get home late and she would be asleep. I had totally missed her day. I watched Lori go to work as an anesthetist at the hospital, and I could tell she hated handing over our baby to a caregiver. I also saw medicine changing, with business driving decision making instead of patient care.

I realized my role was one of reacting to disease rather than creating health, and I decided to change. Despite the protests of many of my physician friends and colleagues, I resigned my role as chairman of my department and director of critical care and moved. I left behind my positions, my house, my income (two of the three extrinsic measures) and moved across the country to live in a little rental house and create what would intrinsically motivate me. Immediately, I had my wife, kids, and life back, and I could follow my aspirations and what really mattered to me.

Although we lived on credit cards for over a year (it was a little scary at times), it was the smartest decision I have ever made because it brought me back to the core of what matters most. I am probably the happiest, most fulfilled and motivated physician in the country as I write these pages because I am helping more people, have more time with my family, and have the opportunity to get up every day and do what is most important to me.

What is it that really truly matters to you? You've got to discover it, uncover it, and go after it. You can decide to do what matters most to you, too. I am not saying you should be as crazy as I was and just burn your ship in the middle of the ocean, but maybe it is time to explore the possibilities.

YOUR FAMILY

If you do not have a family, you can substitute friends for this section.

How would you rate your relationship with
   your family? _____
Are you spending enough time with your family? _____

If no, is it:
Your occupation or other non-negotiable obligations that
   takes you away from them? _____
You are not currently setting aside time for them? _____

If you have children:
Are you attending their events? _____
Involved in their interests? _____
Actively creating memories, moments, and
   adventures? _____
Surprising them with random days or nights out? _____

Family life is something many people take for granted. Yet a healthy life involves nurturing the most important people in our lives in order to continually build our relationships, family, and network of support. Who is on your team? Are you a good team member?

Everyone loves family members and they love us, but because we are obligated to be around them, we generally take them for granted. Our dialogues, conversations, and time together seem to be the first that are put on hold when we are stressed or pressed for time. Often our relational skills are at the lowest level, especially when we are stressed or under crisis. Yet these are the very people that mean the most, will remember us, and pass on our legacy.

Here are some things you can do now to strengthen your bond:

- Look at your calendar and note the dates that matter most to your family members.

- Schedule date night with your significant other, family, and loved ones.

- Consider cutting back on extra projects at work if you need more time.

- Stop volunteering unless you can do it as a family or when they're doing something else.

- When the kids come home from school, stop whatever you are doing and listen, be mindful, and totally present. Do not worry; they will want about four minutes of your time, and then they will be bored with you. You can then go back to whatever important thing you were doing and have only lost minutes. Do not do this and you could lose your child. I read recently that the average time a dad spends with his child is eight minutes a day! How many minutes do you want to spend with yours?

- Plan time together and go to museums, parks, amusement parks, the beach, or a relaxing dinner together.

- Go on camping trips and hikes or work out as a family.

- Take up hobbies you can do as a family.

- Tell jokes; laugh more together.

- Tell them everyday how much you love them, and cuddle and show affection.

- When other family members say something negative to you, let it roll off like water on a duck's back. Let it go. Show kindness and compassion instead for those you truly love. There is probably a frustration they are experiencing and they could use your help. It's probably not about you but really about them, so do not take it personally.

OTHER GENERAL STRESS REDUCERS

- Follow and cultivate your spirituality.

- Enjoy the arts.

- Get into meditation.

- Take up hobbies.

- Get outdoors more.

- Treat your body to massages.

- Laugh more.

- Spend time with friends.

- Play cards.

- Focus on your desired outcomes and avoid negative thoughts.

The more you change your mind-set to develop optimal health, the stronger your mind will become. Health isn't something you can create with one technique or skill. It's a lifelong process of thinking, momentum, and actions. Each day is a new day. If you were discouraged yesterday, it doesn't matter. Move on, let go of that thought, and make a decision to intentionally choose healthy habits today. Start over. Today is the first day of the rest of your life.

As corny as that seems, the health of your body and the health of your mind are connected in a network of daily interactions. Your body supports your mind and your mind supports your body.

You now have the opportunity to create your best health and life, no matter how old you are. Today is the day!

Afterthoughts from the Author

THIS BOOK IS IN MANY WAYS A PREQUEL TO *Dr. A's Habits of Health,* as it is the heady stuff about our minds that many times does not get much attention because of our busy lives. It's a discovery process of how we are thinking about our health, our lives, and ourselves.

Dr. A's Habits of Health is the "how to" create optimal health and provides an in-depth compendium for living a longer, healthier life. But until someone has a deep desire to create optimal health and a strong self-endorsement, they probably won't. What has happened in those four-and-a-half years since I wrote the *Dr. A's Habits of Health* to make me realize that awakening the desire was the first step to discover optimal health? I have observed that people only change if they truly want to change.

I hope this book has awakened your desire to become as optimally healthy as you can possibly become. And may you live the rest of your days in a thriving state of involvement and fulfillment, doing what is most important to you.

Acknowledgments

THERE ARE SO MANY PEOPLE WHO HAVE influenced me in writing this book.

It starts with my wife Lori, who is a master health coach. Traditionally trained as a nurse anesthetist, she embodies all the characteristics that someone who desires to help people help themselves should strive for. Her ability to bring out intrinsic motivation and really understand what people want in their lives has been an inspiration to me, and her practical everyday coaching has helped bring my work to life. Besides, she is my wife, my best friend, and an amazing mother to our two wonderful daughters, Savannah and Erica. They have been so patient and supportive of me through the arduous process of writing this book. I love all my girls so dearly and I am their biggest fan!

And, of course, to my Mom, and to my two other moms, Marilyn and Sharon, I love you!

Next, I would like to thank this incredible team of health coaches who, for over a decade, have spread the outrageous idea that we can create health in our lives, despite this obesegenic world we live in. Their endless work in coaching tens of thousands of people to learn the habits of health has provided a fertile ground for identifying the challenges and obstacles that stand in the way of people discovering their optimal health.

I next want to thank Medifast. For over a decade, this organization has provided the infrastructure necessary to fuel a growing community, focused on health, and has been a great partner in providing the impetus and resources to create a healthier world.

It seems like just yesterday that Brad MacDonald and I sat down and cofounded Take Shape For Life. Brad was a crazy marine (in his own words) and a dreamer physician with the audacious goal that we could change the world. Brad, I know you are watching from a healthier, loftier place, and the legacy is unfolding. Thanks for handing the baton to your brother, Michael, and your daughter Meg, who I have supreme confidence will take the great work we started to new heights, as they support the mission to create a healthier world.

I also want to thank some of the individual people who have influenced my thinking and writing. It starts with my dear friend and mentor Robert Fritz, who, along with my chief in learning critical care, Joe Civetta, has taught me that truth is the most powerful force on earth.

To the health-care professionals who are working alongside us to move medicine into the third era, where we focus on health, not reacting to disease: Dr. Larry Cheskin, Dr. David Katz, Dr. Mark Nelson, Dr. Joe Pecararo, Lori Lynn Andersen RN, Frieda Keller RN, Marsha Hildebrand, Dr. Greg Czer, Dr. Nick Pennings, Dr. Brian Nadolne, Dr. Robert Hambly, Dr. J. C. Doornick, Dr. Ken Kochman, Dr. Ricky Martino, Dr. Dan Van Zandt, Dr. Joseph Fiore, Dr. Cheryl Child, Dr. Deb Sesker, and Dr. Delia Garcia.

I would also like to thank my colleagues in this health movement for all their hard work, especially Dan Bell, Terri and Dave Miller, Greg Rex, Whitney Kell, Dominic and Rita Tarinelli, Margaret Van Houten, Paula Martino, Ron and Chris Goelz, Kim Fiske, Kelly Rife, Lisa and Jaime Castro, Bryan Drollinger, Margaret Hartman, Pat and Stan Staude, and Russ McCann.

Also I would like to acknowledge some recent additions to this mission, Michelle Jones and her amazing support team, and also Tony Jeary,

Brian Biro, David Singer, and Kevin McCarthy, for their belief and undying support of me and our mission.

Then, of course, I want to thank the people who rolled up their sleeves and made this book a reality. Tammy Kling, a fellow Gator, for her tireless work to help hone this book into a finished gem; Seymour Schachter, who created the illustrations and in my opinion is the best illustrator on the planet; and Dede Cummings, who along with Aleta Coursen and Ellen Keelen, brought the tables and charts to life.

And, of course, Dan Ambrosio and the whole DaCapo/Perseus Group for supporting and helping us get out the message, along with the production team at Eclipse Publishing Services: project manager Mark Corsey, copy editor Jane Gebhart, and designer Jill Shaffer.

Last, but certainly not least, to all of you who read this book and make the decision to go for it.

The vision to create a healthy world is alive and growing, and we wish for all the people of the world to join us in creating a healthier, kinder world.

Dr. Wayne Scott Andersen, March 2013

Sample 100-Calorie Fueling Meals

MANY PEOPLE ARE CONFUSED ABOUT what healthy eating really means. There are *three fundamental desired outcomes* if you want to optimize your body and your health:

1. Match your caloric intake to your caloric outtake once you are at a healthy weight, to maintain your optimal weight.

2. Eat mostly foods that optimize your body's functions.

3. Avoid most foods that hurt your body's functions.

Eating three one-hundred-calorie fueling meals and three smaller meals every three hours using portion control and low-glycemic food is a great strategy. The following pages provide some sample fueling suggestions.

Sample Fueling Breaks

Meal replacements make excellent fueling breaks and assure that you're getting a 100-calorie, low-glycemic, nutrient-dense healthy food source.

- Cheese and tomato. One portion (size of two AA batteries) of natural cheese such as cheddar or Monterey Jack with one sliced tomato.
- Endive and tuna salad. One endive leaf with one tablespoon tuna salad, prepared with hummus in place of mayonnaise. Mediterranean Delights makes delicious, organic, low-fat hummus in flavors like tomato basil, and low-glycemic endive makes a handy container for the tuna salad.
- 3 oz mixed nuts (a small handful)
- 10 almonds and celery stick
- 29 pistachios
- 12 cashews
- 20 peanuts
- 2 tbsp sesame seeds
- 4 Brazil nuts. Great for getting your selenium!
- ½ sliced apple with 3 walnuts
- ½ apple with 2 tsp natural peanut butter. Make sure it's all-natural peanut butter: just peanuts and salt.
- ½ cup fresh strawberries with 2 tbsp light whipped topping
- 1 cup fresh cherries
- 1 medium apple
- ½ cup blueberries (high glycemic) or strawberries (lower glycemic) with a dollop of yogurt
- 1 orange
- 1 pear
- ½ peach with 2 tbsp yogurt
- 2 cups raspberries
- 30 raisins
- Fresh veggie mix. 1 cup broccoli, red pepper, cauliflower with 1 tbsp low-fat ranch dressing.
- 6 pieces basil, sliced tomato, and hummus. My wife Lori's creation: put a dab of hummus and tomato on top of a basil leaf—delightful!
- Herbal lentils and one tomato
- Celery sticks with 1 tbsp natural peanut butter
- 1 cup fresh spinach salad with olives
- ¼ cup egg salad with lettuce or endive
- Half small avocado
- Cauliflower (size of paperback)
- 1 cup tomato and cucumber soup
- ¼ cup guacamole. Combine avocado, tomato, lime juice, and hot pepper to taste.
- Basil, tomato, and hummus (1 tomato)
- Grilled portobello mushroom sprinkled with cheese
- 5 cherry tomatoes with one portion cheddar cheese (size of two AA batteries)
- ½ cup endive and cottage cheese spread. In a food processor or

Sample Fueling Breaks

blender, mix cottage cheese, red pepper, fresh parsley, chives, and chopped jalapeno. Spread on endive.

- Eggplant pizza slice. Sprinkle a slice of eggplant with oregano and roast. Melt cheese on top.
- 1 cup vegetarian chili
- ½ cup edamame (soybeans)
- Half red bell pepper dipped in 3 tbsp hummus
- ½ cup cucumber slices
- 1 large dill pickle
- 1 carambola (starfruit)
- 2 cups baby carrots
- 3 celery sticks with 1 tsp natural peanut butter
- ¼ cup hummus and avocado dip with 3 celery stalks
- 1 cup mashed lentils and tomatoes
- Vegetables and dip. Choose either ½ cup cucumber slices, 6 celery sticks, 6 slices red pepper, or ½ cup raw broccoli florets and dip into 2 oz fat-free, sugar-free ranch dressing.
- 1 cup bean and chickpea salad. Toss diced celery, green pepper, cooked red beans, cooked chickpeas, and fresh parsley together with low-calorie balsamic vinaigrette.
- ⅓ cup low-fat cottage cheese with 4 olives
- Yogurt with ¼ cup berries. Yoplait Light plain yogurt is a great choice.

- ½ cup cottage cheese and ½ medium tomato
- 1 Yoplait Light Smoothie
- ½ cup low-fat cottage cheese with 5 strawberries
- 1 serving of string cheese
- 3 oz frozen nonfat yogurt
- 1 square 70% or higher dark chocolate with 5 almonds
- 1 whole deviled egg. Cut a hard-boiled egg in half, mix the yolk with hummus, and fill the egg.
- 1 cup of soup (cream of tomato, cream of chicken, chicken noodle, or vegetable)
- 1 slice Wasa crispbread with 1 oz smoked salmon
- 1 slice whole-grain bread (such as Fiber for Life) with 2 oz fat-free turkey breast
- ½ cup couscous with celery sticks
- 4 slices Melba toast
- 1 slice Wasa crispbread and ½ sliced tomato

Once you've reached a healthy weight, you can add these to the list as well:

- 1 cup fresh mango
- 1 cup cantaloupe
- 1 medium banana
- 28 grapes

This list should help you get started on ideas for your own small meals. Remember, each one should be low glycemic and no higher than 100 calories.

Notes

LETTER FROM DR. A

1. The doctor of the future will give no medicine, but will interest his patients in the care of the human frame, in diet, and in the cause and prevention of disease. —Thomas Edison, 1903

    As quoted in "Wizard Edison" in *The Newark Advocate*, January 2, 1903.

CHAPTER 1

1. In an article in the *New York Times*, writer Michael Moss described the science behind the addictive attributes of junk food.

    NYTimes.com: The Extraordinary Science of Addictive Junk Food, February 24, 2013, http://www.nytimes.com/2013/02/24/magazine/the -extraordinary-science-of-junk-food.html?pagewanted=all&_r=0.

2. Unfortunately, over a decade later, the progression of obesity and poor health has advanced unabated.

    From Michael Moss, *Salt Sugar Fat: How the Food Giants Hooked Us* (New York: Random House, 2013).

3. The fallout is that over seventy million people in the United States are insulin resistant, and encountering metabolic syndrome.

    U.S. News and World Report, September 5, 2005.

"In the United States, an estimated 60 to 70 million individuals are affected by insulin resistance. Statistics report that more than 40% of individuals older than 50 years may be at risk for insulin resistance; however, it can affect anyone at any age." *Pharmacy Times*, October 5, 2012.

4. The American Academy of Neurology announced in October 2012 that physical activity is even more important than mental activity for the brain, even more so than brainteasers, socialization, or crossword puzzles, in terms of cognitive function.

   Daily physical exercise may benefit health, and reduce stress and the risk of Alzheimer's disease, even in people over the age of 80. Study published in the April 18, 2012, online issue of *Neurology*, the medical journal of the American Academy of Neurology.

CHAPTER 3

1. America's health care system is neither healthy, caring, nor a system.
   —Walter Cronkite

   Walter Cronkite (1993), quoted in review of: Norwick R. M. (2004). American Indian Health: Innovations in Health Care, Promotion, and Policy. *J Health Care Poor and Underserved* 15, 493–494.

2. United States is ranked 37th in terms of health among the 191 members of the World Health Organization, and 72nd in terms of overall level of health.

   World Health Organization report 2000.

3. The patient should be made to understand that he or she must take charge of his own life. Don't take your body to the doctor as if he were a repair shop.

   Personal conversation with Dr. Regestein who states the quote comes from a 2010 Reuters interview. Quentin Regestein, Associate Professor of Psychiatry, Harvard Medical School; Associate Psychiatrist, Department of Psychiatry, Brigham and Women's Hospital.

CHAPTER 4

1. Hans Selye, a Hungarian endocrinologist, uncovered the deleterious effects of chronic stress on our bodies. His research revealed that an overstimulated autonomic nervous system leads to a plethora of long-term negative effects on health.

   Hans Selye, *The Stress of Life* (McGraw-Hill Education, 1978).

2. Australia on August 12, 2012, that upheld the constitutionality of tobacco laws.

> Repackaging Cigarettes — Will the Courts Thwart the FDA? Ronald Bayer, Ph.D., Lawrence Gostin, J.D., and Daniel Marcus-Toll, M.S. *N Engl J Med* 2012; 367:2065–2067.

3. Since 1950, death from cardiovascular disease has been reduced approximately 65 percent.

> U.S. Department of Health and Human Services Centers for Disease Control and Prevention, National Center for Health Statistics report; July 2011.

CHAPTER 5

1. The only way to keep your health is to eat what you don't want, drink what you don't like, and do what you'd rather not. —Mark Twain

> Mark Twain, from *Following the Equator*, 1897.

CHAPTER 6

1. A healthy outside starts from the inside. —Robert Urich

> brainyquote.com.

2. Once again, there is a reason why 85 percent of people who go on a diet to lose weight gain it back within two years.

> Long-Term Persistence of Hormonal Adaptations to Weight Loss. Priya Sumithran, M.B., B.S., Luke A. Prendergast, Ph.D., Elizabeth Delbridge, Ph.D., Katrina Purcell, B.Sc., Arthur Shulkes, Sc.D., Adamandia Kriketos, Ph.D., and Joseph Proietto, M.B., B.S., Ph.D. *N Engl J Med,* October 27, 2011.

CHAPTER 7

1. Motivation is what gets you started. Habit is what keeps you going. —Jim Rohn

> Jim Rohn, *7 Strategies for Wealth & Happiness* (Roseville, CA: Prima Publishing, 1996).

CHAPTER 8

1. As long as we are persistent in our pursuit of our deepest destiny, we will continue to grow. We cannot choose the day or time when we will fully bloom. It happens in its own time. —Denis Waitley

> www.waitley.com

CHAPTER 9

1. Life expectancy would grow by leaps and bounds if green vegetables smelled as good as bacon. —Doug Larson

   Victoria Boutenko, *Green for Life* (Berkley, CA: North Atlantic Books).

2. A risk-free life is far from a healthy life. —Deepak Chopra

   The Real Secret to Staying Healthy for Life (Part 1), Huffpost Healthy Living, July 30, 2012; http://www.huffingtonpost.com/deepak-chopra/healthy -lifestyle_b_1694029.html.

CHAPTER 10

1. The awareness that health is dependent upon habits that we control makes us the first generation in history that to a large extent determines its own destiny. —Jimmy Carter

   Jimmy Carter, *Everything to Gain: Making the Most of the Rest of Your Life* (New York: Random House, 1995).

2. You've got bad eating habits if you use a grocery cart in 7-Eleven. —Dennis Miller

   standupcomedyportal.com, The Dennis Miller Show.

3. Albert Bandura of Stanford University did some powerful research on behavior modification.

   Albert Bandura, *Social Learning Theory* (New York: General Learning Press, 1977).

4. The *New England Journal of Medicine* in July 2007 published a social study that confirmed the spread of obesity through associations, even if the relationships were not in the same geographical surroundings.

   The Spread of Obesity in a Large Social Network over 32 Years, Nicholas A. Christakis, M.D., Ph.D., M.P.H., and James H. Fowler, Ph.D. *N Engl J Med* 2007; 357:370–379.

5. In an Australian study, researchers found that couples who changed their behavior as a team were more successful than people going it alone.

   An Innovative Program for Changing Health Behaviours. *Asia Pac J Clin Nutrition* 2002; 11:S586–S597.

6. Also a British study of almost 1500 couples participating in a lifestyle intervention program to reduce the risk of heart disease found that those who benefited the most had partners who also benefited the most.

Changes in Coronary risk and coronary risk factor levels in couples following lifestyle intervention. British Family Heart Study. *Arch Fam Med.* 1997; 6:354–360.

7. A study from the *Annals of Internal Medicine* compared three approaches to lifestyle intervention for producing weight loss in diabetic patients.

   The Effect of Metformin and Intensive Lifestyle Intervention on The Metabolic Syndrome: The Diabetes Prevention Program Randomized Trial, Trevor J. Orchard, M.D.; Marinella Temprosa, M.S.; Ronald Goldberg, M.D.; Steven Haffner, M.D.; Robert Ratner, M.D.; Santica Marcovina, Ph.D., D.Sc.; Sarah Fowler, Ph.D.; *Ann Intern Med.* April 19, 2005.

8. When I coach people through the process of reducing stress, I give them a technique called the relaxation response. This technique was developed by Dr. Herbert Benson at Harvard and involves teaching the neocortex to relax.

   Herbert Benson, Miriam Z. Klipper, *The Relaxation Response* (New York: HarperCollins, 2001).

9. A recent study shows that mindfulness meditation dramatically lowers the inflammatory markers of stress and is an important exercise to protect our bodies.

   Mindfulness meditation techniques designed to reduce emotional reactivity also reduce post stress inflammatory responses and might be useful in chronic inflammatory conditions such as rheumatoid arthritis, psoriasis, inflammatory bowel disease, and asthma, according to a study by Melissa A. Rosenkranz, Ph.D., and colleagues at the University of Wisconsin-Madison, Center for Investigating Healthy Minds in the Waisman Center, *University of Wisconsin News*, 2013.

   The mindfulness-based approach to stress reduction may offer a lower-cost. *Brain, Behavior, and Immunity*, 2013; 27:174 DOI: 10.1016/j.bbi.2012.10.013.

CHAPTER 11

1. Things start out as hopes and end up as habits. —Lillian Hellman.
   Thinkexist.com.

2. A recent study by the Cooper Institute showed a dramatic reduction in dementia later in life for those who were fit in their fifties.

   The Association Between Midlife Cardiorespiratory Fitness Levels and Later-Life Dementia: A Cohort Study. Laura F. DeFina, M.D.; Benjamin L. Willis, M.D., M.P.H.; Nina B. Radford, M.D.; Ang Gao, M.S.; David

Leonard, Ph.D.; William L. Haskell, Ph.D.; Myron F. Weiner, M.D.; and Jarett D. Berry, M.D., M.S. *Ann Intern Med.* 2013; 158:162–168, 312–314.

3. A recent study reinforces the power of using visual images, such as an optimal health story board, in improving the health of very overweight children.

   A Picture May Be Worth a Thousand Texts: Obese Adolescents' Perspectives on a Modified Photovoice Activity To Aid Weight Loss. Susan J. Woolford, M.D., M.P.H., Shahla Khan, B.A., Kathryn L.C. Barr, M.P.H., Sarah J. Clark, M.P.H., Victor J. Strecher, Ph.D., and Kenneth Resnicow, Ph.D. *Childhood Obesity*, June 2012; Volume 8, Number 3. DOI: 10.1089/chi.2011.0095.

4. An estimated 45.3 million people, or 19.3% of all adults (aged 18 years or older), in the United States smoke cigarettes.

   Centers for Disease Control and Prevention. Vital Signs: Current Cigarette Smoking Among Adults Aged ≥ 18 Years—United States, 2005–2010. *Morbidity and Mortality Weekly Report* 2011; 60(33):1207–1212 [accessed January 24, 2012].

5. Cigarette smoking is the leading cause of preventable death in the United States.

   Centers for Disease Control and Prevention. Annual Smoking-Attributable Mortality, Years of Potential Life Lost, and Economic Costs—United States, 1995–1999. *Morbidity and Mortality Weekly Report* 2002; 51(14):300–303 [accessed January 24, 2012].

6. Cigarette smoking . . . accounting for approximately 443,000 deaths, or 1 of every 5 deaths, in the United States each year.

   Centers for Disease Control and Prevention. Annual Smoking-Attributable Mortality, Years of Potential Life Lost, and Productivity Losses—United States, 2000–2004. *Morbidity and Mortality Weekly Report* 2008; 57(45):1226–1228 [accessed 2012 Jan 24].

7. Cigarette smoking . . . accounting for approximately 443,000 deaths, or 1 of every 5 deaths, in the United States each year.

   U.S. Department of Health and Human Services. The Health Consequences of Smoking: A Report of the Surgeon General. Atlanta: U.S. Department of Health and Human Services, Centers for Disease Control and Prevention, National Center for Chronic Disease Prevention and Health Promotion, Office on Smoking and Health, 2004 [accessed 2012 Jan 24].

CHAPTER 12

1. A diet is a plan, generally hopeless, for reducing your weight, which tests your willpower but does little for your waistline. —Herbert B. Prochnow

   Toastmasters

2. The notes section at the end of the book has further reading about how discovering and reaching optimal health can help you live a longer healthier life.

   Recent literature is filled with discussions of the importance of reaching a healthy weight and adopting a healthy lifestyle. Below are four very powerful large studies which leave no doubt that reaching a healthy weight and learning the habits of health can profoundly affect our health and our lives.

   - Actual causes of death in the United States. McGinnis JM, Foege WH. US Department of Health and Human Services, Washington, DC. *JAMA* 1993; 270(18):2207–2212.

   - Healthy living is the best revenge: findings from the European Prospective Investigation into Cancer and Nutrition—Potsdam study. Ford ES, Bergmann MM, Kröger J, Schienkiewitz A, Weikert C, Boeing H, Division of Adult and Community Health, National Center for Chronic Disease Prevention and Health Promotion, Centers for Disease Control and Prevention, Atlanta, GA. *Arch Intern Med.* 2009; 169(15):1355–1362. DOI: 10.1001/archinternmed.2009.237.

   - Influence of individual and combined health behaviors on total and cause-specific mortality in men and women: the United Kingdom health and lifestyle survey. Kvaavik E, Batty GD, Ursin G, Huxley R, Gale CR. *Arch Intern Med.* 2010; 170(8):711–718. DOI: 10.1001/archinternmed .2010.76.

   - Following cancer prevention guidelines reduces risk of cancer, cardiovascular disease, and all-cause mortality. McCullough ML, Patel AV, Kushi LH, Patel R, Willett WC, Doyle C, Thun MJ, Gapstur SM. *Cancer Epidemiol Biomarkers Prev.* 2011; 20(6):1089–1097. DOI: 10.1158/1055-9965.EPI-10-1173. Epub April 5, 2011.

CHAPTER 13

1. Tell me what you eat and I will tell you what you are. —Anthelme Brillat-Savarin

   Physiologie du Gout, ou Meditations de Gastronomie Transcendante, 1826.

2. Studies from Harvard and UCLA suggest that meal replacement may be helpful for long-term maintenance.

> Research Shows How People Lost More Weight on a Meal Replacement Diet than Counterparts, from Clinical Capsules: Count Those Calories (Brief Article). *Family Practice News*, December 1, 2003.

> Long-term use of a premeasured meal-replacement plan appears to be an effective tool for weight-loss maintenance, Dr. George L. Blackburn reported in a poster presented at the annual meeting of the North American Association for the Study of Obesity.

CHAPTER 14

1. A man's health can be judged by which he takes two at a time—pills or stairs. —Joan Welsh

> Iwise.com.

2 Dr. James A. Levine at Mayo Clinic has extensively studied NEAT.

> James A. Levine, Move a Little, Lose a Lot: New N.E.A.T. Science Reveals How to Be Thinner, Happier, and Smarter (New York: Crown Archetype, 2009. *Best Pract Res Clin Endocrinol Metab*. 2002; 16(4):679–702.

CHAPTER 15

1. [A]n average woman should have about twenty more minutes of sleep a night than a man.

> 1998 National Sleep Foundation poll, women and sleep, http://www .dailymail.co.uk/health/article-2292195/Its-official-Women-ARE -grumpier-men-mornings.html.

EPILOGUE

1. Health is a large word. It embraces not the body only, but the mind and spirit as well . . . and not today's pain or pleasure alone, but the whole being and outlook of a man. —James H. West

> www.totalhealth.bz.

Index

About the Author

ONE OF THE FOREMOST AUTHORITIES IN nutritional intervention and lifestyle management, Dr. Wayne Scott Andersen has devoted his career to forging into new territory in creating optimal health through a comprehensive approach. His insatiable desire to actually help people create health in their lives has put him in position to lead a revolution in health. Unlike those focused on disease or even prevention, Dr. Andersen's innovative approach is to promote real-life ways of helping people break through the logistical and psychological barriers that prevent them from optimizing their health.

He is a best-selling author of the groundbreaking book, *Dr. A's Habits of Health*, and with his second book, *Living a Longer Healthier Life*, has built a lifestyle program that has helped over a hundred thousand people change their perspectives on what it takes to create health in their lives.

Featured on Good Morning America, Dr. Andersen is lecturing internationally on how we can overcome the obesity epidemic and redirect the health-care system to be focused on health.

Dr. A is a driving force in helping move medicine into the third era, where the focus is on partnering with patients to give them the strategies, tools, and the skills to create health instead of react to disease.

Dr. Andersen is very familiar with the undue suffering, loss of lives, and massive costs to individuals and society as a result of an unhealthy lifestyle.

As the tenth board-certified physician in critical care medicine, he helped pioneer the emerging subspecialty of intensive care medicine, serving as director of critical medicine at Grandview Medical Center.

Now as cofounder of Take Shape For Life, Dr. Andersen has built an integrated support system that helps people make the necessary changes in their lifestyles to create optimal health. Using a team approach of health professionals working with health coaches, Dr. Andersen says we can provide leading-edge nutritional solutions, medical support, and the support of caring individuals to foster the necessary one-on-one interaction so vital in changing people's lives. The Take Shape For Life physician-led health network is gathering tremendous momentum. "I am amazed by the power this group of people is having on society. We have a massive epidemic of overweight, unhealthy individuals and I smile every day as we expose more and more people to a real solution that actually works!" says Dr. A.

Dr. Andersen currently lives on the Chesapeake Bay in Annapolis, Maryland, with his wife Lori, a registered nurse who provides nursing support for Take Shape For Life, and is heavily involved in both coaching individuals to optimal health and training coaches to do the same. They have two teenage children, Savannah and Erica.